Health, Technology and Society

Series Editors
Andrew Webster
Department of Sociology
University of York
York, UK

Sally Wyatt
Royal Netherlands Academy of Arts
Amsterdam, The Netherlands

Medicine, health care, and the wider social meaning and management of health are undergoing major changes. In part this reflects developments in science and technology, which enable new forms of diagnosis, treatment and delivery of health care. It also reflects changes in the locus of care and the social management of health. Locating technical developments in wider socio-economic and political processes, each book in the series discusses and critiques recent developments in health technologies in specific areas, drawing on a range of analyses provided by the social sciences. Some have a more theoretical focus, some a more applied focus but all draw on recent research by the authors. The series also looks toward the medium term in anticipating the likely configurations of health in advanced industrial society and does so comparatively, through exploring the globalization and internationalization of health.

More information about this series at
http://www.springer.com/series/14875

Rebecca Lynch · Conor Farrington
Editors

Quantified Lives and Vital Data

Exploring Health and Technology
through Personal Medical Devices

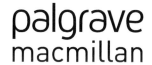

Editors
Rebecca Lynch
London School of Hygiene and Tropical
 Medicine
London, UK

Conor Farrington
School of Clinical Medicine
University of Cambridge
Cambridge, UK

Health, Technology and Society
ISBN 978-1-349-95769-9   ISBN 978-1-349-95235-9   (eBook)
https://doi.org/10.1057/978-1-349-95235-9

This Palgrave Macmillan imprint is published by Springer Nature
The registered company is Macmillan Publishers Ltd.
The registered company address is: The Campus, 4 Crinan Street, London, N1 9XW, United Kingdom

Series Editors' Preface

Medicine, health care and the wider social meaning and management of health are undergoing major changes. In part, this reflects developments in science and technology, which enable new forms of diagnosis, treatment and the delivery of health care. It also reflects changes in the locus of care and burden of responsibility for health. Today, genetics, informatics, imaging and integrative technologies, such as nanotechnology, are redefining our understanding of the body, health and disease; at the same time, health is no longer simply the domain of conventional medicine, nor the clinic. The 'birth of the clinic' heralded the process through which health and illness became increasingly subject to the surveillance of medicine. Although such surveillance is more complex, sophisticated and precise, as seen in the search for 'predictive medicine', it is also more provisional, uncertain and risk laden.

At the same time, the social management of health itself is losing its anchorage in collective social relations and shared knowledge and practice, whether at the level of the local community or through state-funded socialised medicine. This individualisation of health is both culturally driven and state sponsored, as the promotion of 'self-care' demonstrates. The very technologies that redefine health are also the means through which this individualisation can occur—through 'e-health', diagnostic tests and the commodification of restorative tissue, such as stem cells, cloned embryos and so on.

This series explores these processes within and beyond the conventional domain of 'the clinic' and asks whether they amount to a qualitative shift in the social ordering and value of medicine and health. Locating technical developments in wider socio-economic and political processes, each book discusses and critiques recent developments within health technologies in specific areas, drawing on a range of analyses provided by the social sciences.

The series has already published 18 books that have explored many of these issues, drawing on novel, critical and deeply informed research undertaken by their authors. In doing so, the books have shown how the boundaries between the three core dimensions that underpin the whole series—health, technology and society—are changing in fundamental ways.

This new book picks up some of these key themes. By focusing on 'personal medical devices', the editors and contributors explore the ways in which new developments in technology affect how people understand their own bodies, what this means for 'self-care' and how this 'self-care' pervades everyday life. The terms 'personal', 'medical' and 'device', separately and in combination, focus attention on technologies that may be ubiquitously present, in one way or another, in an individual's everyday environment as well as in clinical settings, and whose functions either include, or are entirely devoted to, the diagnosis, monitoring and/or treatment of illness (for 'medical' devices) or the tracking of activity and biometrics (for 'wellness' devices, although these two categories of devices may not be straightforwardly separable). This approach captures devices that are both digital and non-digital in kind, and both medical and wellness in focus. Consequently, a smartphone app or pen and paper diary that an individual carries with them to monitor diet and exercise can be just as much a PMD as the latest digital activity wristband or cutting-edge medical device.

The various contributions to this book demonstrate that personal medical devices (PMDs) reconfigure not only people's health, but also create new socio-material relations between people, friends, colleagues and healthcare providers of different sorts. The volume is divided into four sections. The first provides background to the emergence of PMDs and to different approaches to studying them. The remaining sections address the 'personal', the 'medical' and the 'device', by presenting a rich array of case studies, ranging from ovulation monitors to e-cigarettes to blood pressure monitors.

This new book contributes to one of the series' themes, namely the exploration of recent developments in health technology innovation and how these redefine the relationship between the body and the clinic, between one's own experience and how it compares with the performance of others, via self-tracking of different forms, for example. Contributors also explore how market and regulatory forces are shaping the design, take-up and use of personal medical devices in the workplace. The medical and non-medical uses of such devices pose particular regulatory challenges, not only about how to regulate the devices, but also how these increasingly ubiquitous devices may come to regulate people as patients and as workers.

York, UK   Andrew Webster
Amsterdam, The Netherlands   Sally Wyatt

Acknowledgements

This book arose from conversations between the editors about different approaches taken to technology and health across the social sciences and, as we were both based in a department attached to the clinical school at the University of Cambridge, the degree to which these approaches were accessible to those outside or on the edge of these disciplines. Working on different projects, we also saw interesting potential in examining the intersections between people, health and technology through the consideration of particular medical devices (widely defined), as a way of examining larger questions about understandings and constructions of the body, medicine and technology itself. These conversations led to a symposium, held at the University of Cambridge in September 2014; we are very grateful to Simon Cohn for his support in developing the idea and to the Wellcome Trust for funding the symposium through an Ethics & Society grant (WT104725MA). The chapters in this collection largely result from papers presented at this event. We are extremely grateful for the discussions and comments from those attending the symposium in shaping this collection, particularly Simon Cohn, Catherine Will, Kate Weiner, Flis Henwood, Nick Fox, Giulia Colvolpe Severi and Michael

Hauskeller, as well as those who have contributed to the volume itself. We are grateful too for the assistance of Deborah Lupton, Jeanette Pols and Annemarie Jutel, and to the series editors and Palgrave Macmillan in guiding and enabling us to further develop our ideas as an edited volume. Lastly, we, and the contributors to the volume, would like to thank the individuals with whom we worked to produce these contributions. All interviewees gave permission for their words to be reproduced, and ethical permissions were granted where necessary. We hope this volume contributes to the development of many further conversations in this area.

Contents

Editors and Contributors

About the Editors

Rebecca Lynch is a Research Fellow in Medical Anthropology at London School of Hygiene and Tropical Medicine. She is interested the differing ways in which the body and notions of risk are constructed including through medical technologies, medical practices and moral frameworks. Her approach includes a focus on objects and the material body, and she has undertaken ethnographic fieldwork in Trinidad and the UK. She is a Research Associate at Lucy Cavendish College Cambridge.

Conor Farrington is a Research Associate at the Cambridge Centre for Health Services Research, University of Cambridge School of Clinical Medicine. His research focuses on the medical, sociological and philosophical implications of new medical technologies, especially wearable technologies such as 'artificial pancreas' systems for people with type 1 diabetes.

Contributors

Peta Bush is a Ph.D. Researcher at The Cass, London Metropolitan University. Her research explores design for care of person-centric health artefacts. She is also a designer-maker developing therapeutic jewellery as orthoses using traditional and digital technologies.

Farzana Dudhwala is a Postdoctoral Researcher at the Nuffield Department of Primary Care Health Sciences at the University of Oxford. She specialises in the field of science and technology studies and is especially interested in theories of agency and performativity. In her previous research, Dudhwala studied practices of self-quantification and ethnographically examined the implications of the 'doing' of the self. In her current role, she is again using ethnographic methods, but now to understand how online patient feedback works (or doesn't) within NHS institutions.

Alex Faulkner is Professor in Sociology of Biomedicine & Healthcare Policy in the Centre for Global Health Policy at the University of Sussex, UK. His research interests are in the regulation of novel biomedical technologies and medical devices in the UK/EU and their adoption and non-adoption into healthcare systems. He also undertakes research on bioinformatics policy in India, prostate cancer screening policy and biological therapies in sport.

Ava Hess is an independent scholar who conducted research in support of her contribution to this publication as a graduate student in Visual, Material and Museum Anthropology at the University of Oxford. She is interested in the body both as a means and subject of study, within contexts related to technology, art, or political activism.

Anthony Kent is Professor of Fashion Marketing at Nottingham Trent University and was previously Associate Dean for Research at the London College of Fashion. His current research is in the convergence of digital and physical environments with a focus on fashion retailing, the personalisation of design and fashion and disability.

Mette Kragh-Furbo is a Postdoctoral Research Associate in the DEMAND centre, Lancaster University. Her research focuses on the governance of energy demand in non-domestic environments with a particular focus on energy data practices. In her doctoral research, she studied data practices within consumer genomics.

Adrian Mackenzie (Professor in Technological Cultures, Department of Sociology, Lancaster University) has published work on technology: *Transductions: Bodies and Machines at Speed* (2002); *Cutting Code: Software and Sociality* (2006); *Wirelessness: Radical Empiricism in Network Cultures* (2010); and *Into the Data: An Archaeology of Machine Learning* (2016). He is currently working on the circulation of data-intensive methods across science, government and business in network media. He currently co-directs the Centre for Science Studies, Lancaster University, UK.

Steve Matthewman is Head of Sociology and Criminology at the University of Auckland. Teaching and research interests include science and technology studies, social theory, the sociology of disasters and the sociology of the military. His latest book, *Disasters, Risks and Revelation: Making Sense of Our Times,* was published by Palgrave Macmillan in 2015.

Maggie Mort is Professor in the Sociology of Science, Technology & Medicine at Lancaster University, UK. She has extensive experience in running international interdisciplinary research and was coordinator of the EC FP7 project: Ethical Frameworks for Telecare Technologies for older people at home (EFORTT). She teaches on disaster studies, patient safety and medical uncertainty and supervises doctoral students in the sociology of science and technology. She has published widely from ethnographic research in health, medicine and the implementation of new technologies.

Celia Roberts is Professor in Gender and Science Studies and the Pro-Director of the Centre for Gender and Women's Studies in the Department of Sociology at Lancaster University. She works on sexuality, sex/gender, medicine and science and her most recent book is

Puberty in Crisis: The Sociology of Early Sexual Development (Cambridge UP 2016).

Anna Smajdor is Associate Professor of Practical Philosophy at the University of Oslo. Prior to that, she was Ethics Lecturer at Norwich Medical School, University of East Anglia. Anna's research interests incorporate a range of bioethical themes. She has worked extensively on the ethics of new reproductive technologies and has published widely on medical and research ethics. She is interested in questions concerning the relationship between nature and morality, especially in the context of medicine, scientific research and innovation.

Andrea Stöckl is a medical sociologist/anthropologist at the Norwich Medical School at the University of East Anglia. After finishing degrees in Medical Anthropology and a Ph.D. in Social Anthropology at the University of Cambridge, she focussed her research on the politics of vaccination policies, especially in Europe and in Great Britain, with a focus on women's health issues. Her other interests lie in the ethics of care and the emotional aspects of care. She has also published on controversial surgery on women, such as hymen reconstruction and female genital mutilation. She is interested on the intersections of ethics and sociology of medicine.

Chris Till is a Senior Lecturer in Sociology at Leeds Beckett University whose work focuses on health, technologies, the digital and social theory. He is currently conducting research into the use of self-tracking devices in corporate wellness programmes.

Joann Wilkinson is a Doctoral Researcher at Lancaster University in the Department of Sociology. Her research looks at how women use ovulation biosensing technologies when trying to become pregnant. Key interests include: the body, reproductive technologies, feminism and fertility.

List of Figures

List of Tables

Part I
Introduction

1

Personal Medical Devices: People and Technology in the Context of Health

Conor Farrington and Rebecca Lynch

Technological innovation has always been integral to health and health care, contributing to the development and implementation of new possibilities for medical intervention in diagnostic, therapeutic and preventative modalities. In recent years, however, there has been a notable proliferation of medical technologies tailored to individuals, often drawing on developments in digital technology, and frequently for use outside 'traditional' medical locations. We have termed these technologies 'personal medical devices' (PMDs)—devices that are attached to, worn by, interacted with, or carried by individuals for the purposes of generating biomedical data and/or carrying out medical interventions on the person concerned. Such technologies have become increasingly

C. Farrington (✉)
Cambridge Centre for Health Services Research,
University of Cambridge, Cambridge, UK
e-mail: Cjtf2@medschl.cam.ac.uk

R. Lynch
London School of Hygiene and Tropical Medicine,
University in London, London, UK
e-mail: Rebecca.Lynch@lshtm.ac.uk

© The Author(s) 2018   3
R. Lynch and C. Farrington (eds.), *Quantified Lives and Vital Data*,
Health, Technology and Society, https://doi.org/10.1057/978-1-349-95235-9_1

significant in both clinical and extra-clinical contexts, creating new sites and occasions for intervention, and arguably extending the purview of medicine into other locations and aspects of everyday life. The general (if tentative and uneven) shift towards technological healthcare solutions in wealthy countries reflects the increasing sophistication and miniaturisation of personal devices themselves, in addition to wider shifts towards personalised, patient-centred medicine.

In recent years, policymakers have been increasingly drawn to technological solutions for pressing healthcare challenges, such as those presented by rising levels of multimorbidity and chronic disease in ageing populations. Wearable devices—portable and often digital technologies that individuals attach to their clothing or skin—have frequently been seen as representing the promise of new medical technologies, both within and outside explicitly medical contexts. In 2015, the Medical Director of the English National Health Service (NHS), Bruce Keogh, stated that the NHS will engage in a 'huge rollout' of wearable devices such as wrist-mounted heart monitors and gait-sensing polo shirts as part of a 'revolution in self-care' (Campbell 2015). New initiatives in this context include the NHS Test Beds, which will trial wearable and mobile health technologies for conditions such as diabetes and mental illness (NHS England 2016). Outside clinical settings, data-generating wearable technologies are big business. While phone companies now standardly embed activity monitors and health apps into our smartphones, corporations not only market wearables as useful and fashionable consumer devices (e.g. Apple Watch, Fitbit by Tory Burch), but also increasingly use them to monitor workforce activity and productivity (Rich and Miah 2016; Till, this volume). Consumer use of wearable devices for medical and wellness purposes has risen rapidly in recent years, with UK sales of wearables estimated to reach 5 million units in 2016 (from 3 million in 2015; WearableTech 2016). Groups such as the Quantified Self movement, in which individuals use technology to undertake self-tracking activities to improve daily functioning, reflect growing interest in the use of PMDs to improve wellness and postpone sickness outside clinical arenas (Dudhwala, this volume).

Influenced furthermore by the growing presence of notions of Big Data in public discourse, the burgeoning PMD field is advancing rapidly across multiple domains and disciplines. In fact, this advance is occurring so rapidly that our conceptual and empirical understandings of PMDs—what PMDs 'do' in different locations'—and the wider clinical, social and philosophical implications that may result, often lag behind new technical developments and medical interventions. Experience of previous technologies attests that this state of affairs is by no means unprecedented. When the motor car was introduced to Britain's roads, for instance, a Royal Commission of 1906 (and subsequent parliamentary discussions) focused heavily on the nuisance caused by cars raising clouds of dust by the roadside (Hansard 1908). Other and more serious problems (e.g. accidents, road rage, gridlock, negative impacts on urban design) were either not foreseen or downplayed. As Matthewman (2011: 24) notes, what technology 'actually does' in practice is 'never a final accomplishment; it always remains an ongoing process'. Furthermore, with the digital revolution in computing, and by extension all the areas of life in which computing is relevant, perhaps we are all now 'Sunday drivers', as Jean Baudrillard Baudrillard (Baudrillard 2005: 214) puts it—permanently mystified and baffled by the increasingly complex, powerful, miniaturised, interconnected, and ubiquitous technologies that we increasingly rely upon. As such, it is perhaps unsurprising that scholars have yet to take full account of the manifold complexities of PMD usage in a range of settings.

A key imperative facing academic explorations of PMDs is the need to avoid uncritically embracing (and thus reiterating) either side of the simplistic divide between techno-utopian and techno-dystopian discourses. This duality frequently characterises public discourse around new technologies and encourages views of PMDs as either clinical panacea or Orwellian threat. In order to take a more balanced approach that engages with users' experiences of PMDs in practice, nuanced, critical, and empirically grounded approaches are needed to interrogate and understand emerging issues in this field. This is so both in terms of how people experience the devices themselves—what might be termed the ethnography of technology—and also what these experiences might mean for our wider, sociologico-philosophical understandings of self and society. There is room, that is, for social scientists to stake a claim in this emerging field and to ask important questions neglected by others.

Furthermore, this area also provides much 'meat' for social scientists to chew on, bringing to the fore particular relationships, conceptualisations and socialities, which in turn may impact on how we, and our interlocutors, understand and 'do' health, medicine, and the body. This volume aims to contribute to such work and to illustrate some of the key issues and salient considerations to which future research in this field should attend.

PMDs as Conceptual Starting Point

In drawing together the varied interactions between individuals, technologies and health, we also seek to reflect the diversity of these devices and some of the different disciplinary approaches to technology itself, while still holding together a central cohesive narrative that runs through these. We do this by drawing upon the concept of PMDs to foreground discussion on the intersection between people, technologies and health, and particularly those devices focused on/personalised for the individual to contribute to their well-being. The development of new concepts, such as our notion of PMDs, often contributes to significant advances in particular fields, as seen, for instance, in Donna Haraway's seminal exploration of the cyborg (Haraway 1991) and, more recently, in Ulucanlar et al. (2013) adumbration of the notion of 'technology identities'. Such concepts facilitate both *originality* (in terms of facilitating new and innovative ways of thinking about things) and *utility* (in terms of providing a central analytical focus for empirical investigations; Corley and Gioia 2011). Through the concept of PMDs, we aim in this volume to enable the development of both incremental and revelatory insights by building upon and re-framing research on a range of technologies and in a range of disciplines, while simultaneously facilitating the emergence of new forms of understanding.

The concept of PMDs may be described as a portmanteau concept, bringing together a number of elsewhere separated aspects. We coordinate the terms 'personal', 'medical' and 'device' in order to focus attention on technologies that may be ubiquitously present, in one way or another, in an individual's everyday environment as well as in clinical settings, and whose functions either include, or are entirely devoted to, the diagnosis, monitoring and/or treatment of illness (for 'medical' devices) or the tracking of activity and biometrics (for 'wellness' devices, although these two categories of devices may not be straightforwardly separable). This approach consciously casts a wider net than many analytical approaches, since it includes devices that are both digital and non-digital in kind, and both medical and wellness in focus. Consequently, a smartphone app or pen and paper diary that an individual carries with them to monitor diet and exercise can be just as much a PMD as the latest digital activity wristband or cutting-edge medical device. Furthermore, the concept does not exclude any specific kind of interaction with the body: PMDs can be carried in clothing or baggage, worn on the body and implanted or ingested within it. As such, the silos that tend to characterise existing research on PMDs— e.g. research on wearables, 'insideables' (implantable devices), 'smart' garments, smartphone apps and paper diaries—can be overcome by utilising a concept that unites these seemingly disparate technologies through their shared focus on personal wellness and its obverse, illness. This focus highlights a kinship between PMDs and other, more static and less ubiquitous medical technologies such as MRI scanners, intravenous drips, or even the traditional doctor's stethoscope. However, incorporating devices upon and within the body alters our engagements with technology in potentially different ways by questioning bodily boundaries, moving beyond Cartesian mind–body dualities and raising new issues of surveillance and trust. Thus, our engagements with PMDs proffer a distinctive kind of relationship, more intimate and potentially more angst-ridden, than we may experience with many other kinds of medical technology.

A further characteristic of our approach is a concern to interrogate each dimension of this portmanteau concept, such that 'the personal', 'the medical' and 'the device' each come under scrutiny. The 'personal' nature of such devices is not solely limited to a particular user, for example, since PMDs usage typically relies on a wide range of sociotechnical networks incorporating multiple kinds of actors (e.g. carers, clinicians, policymakers, technologists, designers) and infrastructures (e.g. manufacturing capacities, national electricity supply, telecommunications networks). Similarly, the concepts of 'the medical' and 'the device' are part of wider practices, networks and understandings. As such, the concept of the PMD does not seek to close off, delimit, or—as Steve Matthewman, citing John Law (1992), puts it in this volume—'punctualise' individual PMDs as they are experienced in practice, but rather encourages the critical examination of wider dynamics and networks in addition to the use of PMDs in practice. As such, the concept of PMDs contributes to wider discussions of individual responsibility for health and health care, and medical provision in the context of ageing societies, rising levels of chronic disease and multimorbidity, and budgetary pressures.

New technologies therefore alter not only health but also sociomaterial relations. As the chapters in this volume go on to show, PMDs create new relationships with others—health professionals, employers and peers (including other individuals also using PMDs). They impact on people's relationships with their own bodies and their understandings of health. They construct bodies in different ways—as being knowable through specific forms of data, as bounded in particular ways, as new sites of possible intervention, and as producing and aligning new risks. Understandings of health may relate not only to subjective assessments of individual experiences but also to 'objectively' measured data that may be comparable to previous readings, readings from others or pre-identified norms. These different forms of understandings—measurements and personal feelings or experiences—may be brought together to a greater or lesser extent, working together, contradicting or taking precedence over each other. Indeed, such technologies may create new ways of being through new modes of knowing. While these data might be reflected on locally, shared with friends, family members and/or health professionals, these measurements, and the technologies themselves, may circulate globally and become embedded in micro-dynamics of power (Hardon and Moyer 2014), creating new power relations on a global scale. These raise questions about to whom such data and technologies belong, who decides upon their use, and to whom they are available. Like other aspects of science and medicine, these are not neutral tools.

As such, these technologies and their effects cannot be excluded from social analysis. Previous research by social theorists, including work by Marx and Foucault, has focused on the role of the material in social relations and in creating healthy and productive individuals. In particular, Foucauldian analysis of the hegemonic character of medical technologies and the role of governments in developing personal responsibility for health through such technologies has resulted in a huge body of literature in this field (Hardon and Moyer 2014). More recent work from Science and Technology studies (STS) has incorporated material elements within social analysis and has proved especially influential in pushing forward and developing thinking in this area, as many contributions to this volume attest (e.g. Kragh-Furbo et al., this volume; Dudhwala, this volume; Lynch, this volume; and Faulkner, this volume). Such work can be linked to Latour's call for a richer ethnography, where we might think of 'the social' as being made up of not only people but also 'things' (Latour 2005). He, like other STS theorists, argues that material objects ('non-humans') are so integral to our everyday lives that excluding these limits our social analysis. For Latour, technologies themselves make human society: 'Without technological detours, the properly human cannot exist' (Latour 2002, p. 252). Such a conceptualisation has further implications when we think about bodies, medicine and health. Connected bodies and medical technologies may be hard to disentangle, making it unclear where one ends and the other starts. The notion of health may cut across individual human bodies to encompass the health of objects or things; as Matthewman notes in his introductory paper (this volume), the 'health' and functioning of technology impacts on, and is part of, human health. The health of individuals is reliant on the functioning of non-human objects with which it interacts.

Researching PMDs

This edited collection therefore focuses on the crossing points between technologies, people and health, on the different intersections, relations and constructions that emerge at these crossing points, and on their wider consequences. In the papers that follow, we have drawn together different approaches to investigating this field. The chapters focus on different examples of the many technologies available for different medical purposes and on the varied questions that these raise. Some of these technologies are situated within explicitly medical arenas or are aimed at particular conditions such as type 1 diabetes (e.g. Hess, this volume; Farrington, this volume). Others look at the use of health technologies outside such explicitly medical settings, including use by employers (Till, this volume), interested individuals (Kragh-Furbo et al., this volume; Dudhwala, this volume) and for 'keepsakes' (Smajdor and Stockl, this volume). As previously noted, many of the papers draw on STS approaches in considering the technologies on which they focus. Others are tied to more classic sociological approaches (e.g. Farrington, this volume; Till, this volume), while some come from particular perspectives such as medical ethics (Smajdor and Stockl, this volume) or design (Kent and Bush, this volume). All papers situate and give some description of their approach for readers less familiar with their fields.

In order to keep some central focus within a collection that aims to present different technologies, issues and approaches, all papers concentrate upon the UK context. The UK is a particularly stimulating site for PMD research because of its combination of a national publicly funded health service incorporating cutting-edge technology, a thriving private technology sector with significant innovation occurring in the medical technology sector, and a long history of scientific innovation. The UK also exhibits an interesting policy background, with a strong shift to neoliberalism from the late 1970s and accompanying health reforms incorporating managerialism and New Public Management (Hood 1991; Diefenbach 2009). The contemporary policy scene reinforces the perceived need for technologies such as PMDs in order to ease NHS budget pressures arising from ageing, obesity, chronic diseases and co-morbidity, amidst cuts to social care and other budgets. As such, the UK not only has unique aspects but also exhibits similarities and crossovers with other wealthy contexts such as North America and Europe. Situating the papers within one over-arching context illustrates some of the range of issues and technologies that are present within one complex system.

Nevertheless, the technologies discussed and issues raised in this collection (e.g. regulation of technologies and framing of medical discourse) are of course not restricted within national boundaries. Part of the stories of these technologies, and theoretical approaches to these technologies, are the supranational networks and relationships that are inherent to this field. Data in the chapters may be UK-based, but these also raise issues and debates that are current in many industrial nations where similar technologies are being used (such as the international growth of the Quantified Self movement originally based in California; see Dudhwala, this volume). Genetic testing using 23andMe technology, the Quantified Self movement, corporate monitoring of employees and regulation of medical devices, to use some of the examples in this collection, all have international origins, interconnections and implications. Analysis of wider underlying concepts – such as the limits of 'the medical' and medicalisation of everyday life, the extent to which objects can 'care' and development of discourses on health technology from within science – are discussions which do not limit themselves to a specific UK context.

The book itself builds upon the research papers and interdisciplinary discussions that took place during a Wellcome Trust-funded Symposium on personal medical devices at the University of Cambridge in September 2014. The chapters bring together important new research from a range of cognate disciplines that focus upon the social implications of new technologies, including sociology, science and technology studies (STS), anthropology, philosophy and design studies, in order to explore the significance of PMDs from different perspectives. Reflecting these varied lenses on the same field, data in these chapters are drawn from the different methodologies appropriate to the range of disciplinary approaches involved. These include interviews, participant observation and other ethnographic approaches in addition to analysis of policy, scientific, ethical, medical and design discourses and genealogies of technology and society. By focusing on the personal, medical and device aspects of PMDs and by drawing upon in-depth empirical research in each of these spheres, the chapters draw out some of the complexities of these technologies as they are used for, and impact on, health, exploring the ways in which they might illuminate, make, alter and/or dissect relationships between people, health and technology.

The edited collection is divided into different sections. While this chapter illustrates the growth of and relevance of the field by introducing the concept of PMDs and some of the key issues in this area, the second introductory chapter by Matthewman locates PMDs within the longer history of social theoretical approaches to medical technology. Taken together, these two chapters provide a backdrop against which the various PMD case studies and theoretical approaches can best be appreciated. The next three parts of the book present original research papers on PMDs and have been grouped in sections which focus upon, and re-formulate, questions around 'the personal' (Kragh-Furbo et al.; Hess; Dudhwala), 'the medical' (Farrington, Smajdor and Stockl, Lynch) and 'the device' (Faulkner, Till, Kent and Bush).

The first three research chapters discuss how PMDs raise questions about the body and bodily boundaries, with particular regard to the distinctiveness of the body as an entity separate from the environment with which it interacts. Mette Kragh-Furbo et al. discuss how two particular PMDs—an ovulation monitor and a consumer gene test—produce biosensor data about individuals, and how this in turn produces different bodies and sense of these bodies. Through presentation and analysis of data from web discussion sites, Kragh-Furbo et al. illustrate how people interpret and make sense of the biosensing data that individuals receive from these PMDs. Arguing that it is precisely through interactions on online forums that a 'biosensing body' might be produced, they present discussions, speculations, bodily sensations and artefacts individuals draw on to 'make up' and 'hold together' the biosensing bodies of women trying to conceive and those seeking to understand their genetic risk. These biosensing bodies and their relationships to the PMDs that contribute to them are quite different from the bodies that Ava Hess argues are made through interactions between people with type 1 diabetes and their insulin pumps. For Hess' interlocutors, their pumps are visual and material mediators of their condition, both for themselves and for others. Through displaying, hiding, quieting or bringing to the fore their pumps in different circumstances, different bodies and different diabetes are 'made', becoming quite different things, even for the same interviewee. The ethnography and interviews conducted by Farzana Dudhwala with members of the Quantified Self movement draw on Baradian conceptualisations to discuss how self-quantifying technologies might facilitate new boundaries between 'the self' and 'the body'. As Kragh-Furbo et al. and Hess also imply, Dudhwala does not suggest that technologies provide data about a stable body already in existence and waiting to be measured, but rather that such data 'make' the bodies of those who interact with it. Dudhwala goes further, however, to detail *how* self-quantifying technologies are an inseparable element of the multiple enactments of the self and the body, demonstrating the potential of Karen Barad's theorising to locate and unpick situations where this occurs for her interviewees.

The next section raises questions about 'the medical' and the medical sphere, e.g. what 'counts' as medical, what might medicine undertaken through PMDs 'do' to patients and what might PMDs 'do' and illustrate about medicine itself. Conor Farrington's chapter draws on the experiences of participants in a research trial of an artificial pancreas for pregnant women with type 1 diabetes. Through a practice-based interpretation Weick's theory of 'sensemaking', an approach more commonly found within organisational studies, Farrington explores how data from a clinical trial technology can reconstitute attitudes to self and technology in the context of medicine, both liberating and constraining individuals in different ways. Anna Smajdor and Andrea Stockl present medical ethics perspectives in their discussion of the 'keepsake ultrasound'—i.e. additional scans sought by pregnant women, which are not provided as part of routine medical care. Smajdor and Stockl suggest that these PMDs raise questions about where the medical realm and its moral imperatives may start and end, with implications for arguments about the special positioning of medicine as a discipline. They point out that some PMDs have both medical and non-medical applications, which may impact on monitoring and regulatory oversight. Another story of regulation, or indeed, prohibition, of difficult-to-categorise PMDs is presented in Rebecca Lynch's chapter on public health discourses around e-cigarettes. While e-cigarettes may arguably be used for medical and/or pleasurable purposes, Lynch examines how these are enacted as particular objects within public health debates—as either good or bad, as impacting on individual smoking behaviour in particular ways, and as objects able to be separated from the contexts in which they are used. Through an examination of how public health constructs these as positive or negative 'risky' objects, Lynch argues that some of the unhelpful assumptions embedded within public health science become visible.

The third and last of the sections focuses on questions around 'the device'—e.g. how might new devices be designed and regulated, how might these be used by institutions, who might be the stakeholders, and who is responsible and involved in making key decisions around these? Alex Faulkner examines regulation and adoption of PMDs within and beyond healthcare systems. Drawing on the regulatory context of the UK, including its relationship to the European Union, Faulkner presents two devices that measure and/or monitor blood flow and pressure. He discusses how regulatory frameworks struggle with new technologies and how uncertainties around regulation may impact on the ways in which users and stakeholders understand, evaluate and engage with these technologies. Chris Till's chapter moves us away from the regulation of devices to discussions of how devices might be used by corporations to regulate their staff. Drawing on the work of Deborah Lupton and others, Till argues that companies are increasingly taking an interest in wellness programmes in which their staff are encouraged to use digital self-tracking devices. He argues that such programmes enable a convergence of 'work' and 'health'. In this convergence, increasing physical activity is linked to increased productivity, so that activity becomes an arbiter of a person's moral value. Lastly, Anthony Kent and Peta Bush adopt a design perspective to discuss the interactions between health technologies and design, before discussing the potential for co-design of PMDs by patients and designers. By engaging with the example of orthotic splints, they map designers' historical involvement in the creation of these items and discuss key aspects that designers should keep in consideration, before presenting a case study of participatory design for a more contemporary and aesthetically pleasing kind of splint. Kent and Bush ask us to consider *who* might be involved in the design of PMDs (why not patients themselves?) and *how* PMDs might be designed (why not as pieces of jewellery?). Their chapter invites us to engage, in a very concrete way, with the STS provocation also raised in Matthewman's introductory chapter: these technologies 'could be otherwise'. Finally, we end the collection with concluding remarks by the editors that reflect on the contributions of these chapters and some of the issues they collectively raise.

References

Baudrillard, J. (2005). *The System of Objects* (J. Benedict, Trans.). London: Verso.

Campbell, D. (2015). Prof Bruce Keogh: Wearable technology plays a crucial part in NHS future. Available online at: https://www.theguardian.com/society/2015/jan/19/prof-bruce-keogh-wearable-technology-plays-crucial-part. Accessed September 1, 2016.

Corley, K., & Gioia, D. (2011). Building theory about theory: What constitutes at theoretical contribution? *Academy of Management Review, 36*(1), 12–32.

Diefenbach, T. (2009). New public management in public sector organizations: The dark side of managerialistic 'enlightenment'. *Public Administration, 87*(4), 892–909.

NHS England. (2016). Test Beds. Available online at: https://www.england.nhs.uk/ourwork/innovation/test-beds/. Accessed December 15, 2016.

Hansard. (1908). Motor car legislation. Available online at: http://hansard.millbanksystems.com/lords/1908/jul/29/motor-car-legislation. Accessed December 15, 2016.

Haraway, D. (1991). *Simians, cyborgs, and women: The reinvention of nature*. New York: Free Association Books.

Hardon, A., & Moyer, E. (2014). Medical technologies: Flows, frictions and new socialities. *Anthropology and Medicine, 12*(2), 107–112.

Hood, C. (1991). A public management for all seasons? *Public Administration, 69*, 3–19.

Latour, B. (2002). Technology and morality: The ends of means. *Theory, Culture & Society, 19*(5/6), 247–260.

Latour, B. (2005). *Reassembling the social: An introduction to actor-network theory*. Oxford: Oxford University.

Law, J. (1992). Notes on the theory of the actor-network: Ordering, strategy, and heterogeneity. *Systems Practice, 5*(4), 379–393.

Matthewman, S. (2011). *Technology and social theory.* Basingstoke: Palgrave Macmillan.

Rich, E., & Miah, A. (2016). Mobile, wearable and ingestible health technologies: Towards a critical research agenda. *Health Sociology Review, 26*(1), 84–97.

Ulucanlar, S., Peirce, S., Elwyn, G., & Faulkner, A. (2013). Technology identity: The role of sociotechnical representations in the adoption of medical devices. *Social Science and Medicine, 98,* 95–105.

WearableTech. (2016). Wearable sales in UK to total five million units in 2016. Available online at: http://www.wearabletechnology-news.com/news/2016/may/17/wearables-sales-uk-total-five-million-units-2016/. Accessed December 15, 2016.

2

Theorising Personal Medical Devices

Steve Matthewman

Introduction

The overarching aim of this chapter is to make sense of Personal Medical Devices (Pmds) from a social science perspective. To do this, I consider both the nature of technology and the active role it plays in the construction of self and society. I begin by introducing standard sociological definitions of technology in order to bring conceptual clarity to the subject area. Five are offered: technology as objects, activities, forms of knowledge, modes of organisation and their combination within complex systems. Having said what technology *is*, I go on to note the issues that preoccupy theorists of technology today. I examine the politics of technology, technology's place within power relations, and its role in both personal and collective well-being. This forms part of a broader consideration of what technologies, PMDs included, *do*.

S. Matthewman (✉)
University of Auckland, Auckland, New Zealand
e-mail: s.matthewman@auckland.ac.nz

© The Author(s) 2018
R. Lynch and C. Farrington (eds.), *Quantified Lives and Vital Data*,
Health, Technology and Society, https://doi.org/10.1057/978-1-349-95235-9_2

This is amplified in the following section, which is devoted to the notion of non-human agency. Drawing on actor-network theory, I note four senses in which technologies can be regarded as actors: I argue that technologies make society possible, function as mediators of our world, perform moral and political functions and gather actors from other times and places. The fourth section engages with current debates around technologies and humanity: do technologies enhance or diminish humanity? The fifth section continues this theme: it looks at the ways in which technologies reconfigure identities, roles and social relations. The sixth section discusses the unintended consequences of personal medical devices. These novel vulnerabilities include powerful new forms of surveillance, the literal possibility of 'life hacking', and reliance upon critical (and very often frail) infrastructures. While these technologies open up a new 'biological' frontier operating between metabolism and mechanism, PMDs map onto old technological impulses to extend human forces and senses, and to help us operate competently in the world. Consequently, I urge us to think of these technologies as prostheses.

Defining Technology: Going Beyond the Thing Itself

This chapter draws on current technological scholarship as a way to both theorise PMDs and discuss the sociological issues and debates that arise from their use. I begin by defining technology. The simplest way to define technology is as objects, which now need to be considered as virtual as well as actual. We should also remember that these objects may be fixed or in flux; software, for example, which helps code ever-greater areas of social life, is virtual, and it tends to upgrade continually. We also need to think about technology as activities (MacKenzie and Wajcman 1985, p. 3). Technologies are normally produced and utilised to create certain effects. In order for these to be realised, we need to know how to use them. This takes us into the realm of technique, which entails right knowing and right doing. Even the simplest tool is useless in the hands of an unskilled user. Three different levels of technology—object, activities and techniques—have been identified, but it is important to remember that they all combine in use. So, for example, you are reading this book. Reading is the activity, and the book is the object, but it relies on technique-related knowledge too, in this case a working knowledge of the English language. A fourth way of seeing technology is as modes of social organisation (Winner 1977, p. 12). This is a necessary addition, for we live in a world in which complex socio-technical systems inform everything that we do.

The notion of the socio-technical system may be invoked to capture our reality and thus to theorise technology properly. We might think of 'a' motor vehicle, but in order for it to operate unproblematically, we require a well-functioning socio-technical system to support it. This system involves such things as roads, signage, street lighting, policing, fuelling and servicing. This in turn relies upon such things as the energy and insurance industries, car manufacturers and numerous regulatory agencies of the state.

The same point holds for PMDs. When we look at 'a' device, we end up with a socio-technical system. All the definitions of technology that have been identified come into play. A single device is never just the thing itself; rather, it is composed of multiple components (hardware and software), practices, knowledges, authorities and organisations. This alignment of a large array of actors is necessary to manufacture the device and manage it, the patient, their records, the medical issue the PMD seeks to resolve and so forth. A network is required to select, fit and configure the PMD, to ensure proper monitoring and use, and to provide follow-up, repair or replacement. The first substantive point is therefore somewhat obvious: the theorising of PMDs can never simply focus on the thing itself as an isolated technology. To do so would be to 'punctualise' the technology, as John Law (1992, p. 385) puts it, which is to say it would essentially abstract the PMD from the networks that produce, support and regulate it. Punctualisation mistakes technology for a single thing, when in reality it is composed of numerous parts (and systems). Following actor-network theory and social thinking's general turn to technology, it is now commonplace to see the big picture, to think about how technologies and other agents are something more than the sum of their parts and to note their connections. This involves locating them within (often very complex) interactive systems and seeing how they are enacted by the networks that sustain them.

In the case of PMDs, complexity exists in their internal components, their bodily connections and their linkages to external systems of maintenance and monitoring. (And we have yet to note the infrastructures that provision energy and communication: power generation systems and the Internet. I note some issues relating to this in the fifth section.) The thing itself may be highly complex, but it is also located upon or within the most complex organic being that exists, and there remains the possibility, at some stage at least, that it will involve a raft of experts within the most complex organisation we have ever created: the hospital (Drucker 2006, p. 54).

Theorising Technology: Five Key Themes

Engagement with the major themes in technological theorising helps us to conceptualise PMDs and to think about the complexities that present themselves when we study them. Here, I suggest that we pay serious attention to the politics of technology (as it relates to form and function); in other words, when thinking about PMDs, we need to think about how, for whom and on what terms they work. Similarly, we need to be mindful of the symbolic and practical elements of these PMDs in order to appreciate what they mean at an individual and collective level.

To begin with, all artefacts have politics. I use 'politics' to refer to the operations of power: the ability to control, regulate, settle outcomes and order others. Artefacts are political in two specific senses. The first is in what might be called an *intrinsic* politics: how technologies like PMDs come to appear and perform in the ways that they do. This takes us to the literature on the social construction of technology (SCOT) and critiques of the notion of 'pure' technology (Bijker 2010). Against such notions, these sociologists stress the *contingency* of technology. John Law and Wiebe Bijker (1992, p. 3) remind us that 'they [i.e. technologies] could be otherwise': the reason being that they are the outcome of compromise. There are competing interests in play, between designers, engineers, manufacturers, marketers, accountants and so on. Take a hypothetical PMD: a designer will be interested in aesthetics, an engineer in how things will work and how materials will perform, while an accountant is interested in how much it all costs. These competing interests can conflict. Some positions win out over others. Here, it should be noted that different stakeholders have different vested interests, and they may well envisage very different types of end user. And when it comes to medical devices, there is considerable debate as to what constitutes a user (see Shah and Robinson 2008).

Then, there are what might be called the *extrinsic* politics of artefacts. Technologies are always designed to do certain things: to help or hinder, to liberate or control and to enable or constrain. Technologies channel action: they permit some behaviours but prevent others. As such, they have a morality to them (Latour 2002a). Sociologically, this brings up numerous questions relating to power, such as what is being decided, and by whom (Pfaffenberger 1992)? Which groups and individuals are advantaged, which disadvantaged, and with what consequences?

The second theme flows on from the first. If technologies shape behaviour, if they have a role in constraining, affording and generally shaping our conduct, then they have an expressly political function. Heed must be paid to the materiality of power, the ways in which power works through objects and organisations (I discuss this in more detail in Matthewman 2011, pp. 70–91). Langdon Winner (1980, p. 128) is insightful here. He concludes that technologies are ways of structuring the world and that divisive or unifying issues are settled both in the formal realm of politics proper and informally through technology, 'in tangible arrangements of steel and concrete, wires and transistors, nuts and bolts'. Winner wants us to think of technologies as new forms of social power, and like those older orderings, as the equivalent of legislative acts.

But in technology, as in formal politics, settlement is only ever a temporary accomplishment. Do today's technologies ever stabilise? Mobile phones originally projected voices. Then, they started to send text. Now, they take photographs, play music, relay moving images, store data and surf the web (Khoo 2005). It should also be acknowledged that stability, when it does emerge, requires ongoing effort. For this reason, Bruno

Latour (2005, p. 143) says that 'work-net' might be a preferable term to 'network' because it foregrounds the labour involved in successfully tying people, institutions and technologies together.

The third theme is subjectivity and technology. If a complex area is reduced to a single question, it can be posed thus: to what extent do technologies make us? How are humans shaped, informed or—thinking about pharmaceuticals and PMDs—even *performed* by technologies of various types? The notion of performance came to prominence through posthuman scholarship, which heralded a move away from representational modes of analysis that merely described reality. In contrast, posthumanist accounts look to explore the ways in which reality is achieved, how it is made in practice and how the world is constructed (Barad 2003, p. 802). This helped bring new attention to the place of technology within explanatory schema. Social theory had tended to regard technology as passive. It was largely given a symbolic role. The posthumanist turn helped stress the material properties of technologies and their ability to exert agency. What sort of person are you, say, minus mobile devices, access to social networking sites or various medicines? (I will return to these issues in the following section on technology and mediation.)

Technological use beyond narrowly instrumental purposes should also be signalled. Technologies can be freighted with symbolism, as earlier theorising has noted. Any watch will mark time, but a luxury watch simultaneously marks status. Technologies charm and are used for a variety of reasons, not all of which are narrowly functional (e.g. emotional appeal or aesthetic quality). Many devices, some PMDs included, are marketed on the twin promises of fashion and fun.

Notions of personhood have always been technologically inflected. The emergence of Web 2.0 produced websites stressing 'writable' user-generated content, social networking, simplicity of use and ease of interaction with other technologies and systems. Here, Facebook is a good example. In contrast to the 'readable' information portals of Web 1.0 like personal web pages, Web 2.0 sites emphasise active use over passive consumption and cooperation over control. These platforms have in turn enabled Health 2.0. This refers to products, services and information relating to health–care workers, patients and researchers, and includes such things as online patient communities and telemedicine. They provide new outlets to express feelings, find community, seek medical advice and exchange information. The proliferation of Web 2.0, mobile technologies and PMDs has also served to further blur the subject/object, self/social, private/public, individual/environment distinctions upon which classical social analysis was founded. Indeed, thanks to such technologies, theorists have announced new ways of being, heralding such things as the emergence of a networked self (Rotman 2008), tethered self (Turkle 2006) and quantified self (Lupton 2013).

This leads into our fourth theme: technology and society. If technology has an important role to play in the formation of individual subjectivity, and in the creation of social selves; if technology channels individual and collective action; if it acts, and if it is implicated in power relations, then it plays important roles *within* society. After all, we relate with, to and through technologies. It is within us (in thought, in some PMDs, through vaccinations), and on us (as contact lenses, clothing, glasses and hearing aids); it exists through us (in language, gesture and technique) and around us (as pills, ambulances and hospitals). Just as technologies play a crucial role in the construction of individual subjects, they also play their part in the construction of society. Early sociology proffered the notion of *social* construction. It suggested that society was 'built' on moral orders and shared social bonds. Contemporary sociology suggests that we take notions of construction more literally. It stresses material properties instead of social projections. It looks at the ways in which society is built, secured and transformed *with* technologies.

The fifth theme is non-human agency. Thinking about the materiality of power, and debates relating to technology's role in the maintenance of social order, forces us to think about what it is that technologies actually *do*. To what extent can they be said to *act?* To answer this, we must trace their effects. This will allow us to assess the ways in which they challenge or contribute to the order of things and to human being. Winner (1977), for instance, suggests that we think about technologies as forms of life. In the following section, I further develop the theme of technological agency by discussing technology's role as mediator. In other words, technologies are shown to materially alter our existence in the world.

Non-human Agency: The Mediating Role of Technology

From the previous section, it can be seen that technologies clearly do things: they channel action, perform political functions and play a part in individual and group identities. Scholars have recognised this. Technologies are no longer 'the missing masses' of social theory, relegated to merely symbolic value (Latour 1992). Matter now matters (Connor 2008). The non-humans have been let in. In this section, I ask: what exactly do they do? How do they exert agency? To clarify, Edwin Sayes (2014) distils decades of the teachings of actor-network theory down to four distinct ways in which technologies actively contribute to social life.

First, technology should be seen as the condition for the possibility of society. This was our closing point in the previous section. Technologies help make society possible; they give it its sturdiness, making social life both stable and predictable. Bruno Latour (2002b, p. 10) writes: 'It is only because there exist *long lasting physical … structures such as buildings, houses, paintings, large stones* etc. that it is possible to entertain at all the notion of a society overarching individual and local interactions. Without the existence of a material artefactual world of things', he says, 'it would almost be impossible for us, anatomically modern humans, to think at all about society'. As we will shortly see, this statement does not only apply to modern humans. As a species, we have always evolved with, and been enhanced by, our technologies. There has never been a time when human beings have been without technological assistance. Nor does Latour's point apply to artefacts and architectures alone; it also holds for our other defining elements of technology: institutions and organisations.

It is possible to observe group organisation that is socially and politically complex minus tools or technology of any type. Under such conditions, relations are friable, and consequently in need of constant maintenance and repair. But such observations are not made of humans. Does this mean that traditional sociology is useless? No, answer actor-network theorists, it is perfectly adequate for baboons (Callon and Latour 1981). The first thing that technologies do, then, is stabilise society.

Second, technologies do not just transport or channel action—they do something more. They materially alter associations and interactions. They have effects of their own. Technologies mediate between the physical world and culture, between matter and meaning. Thus, says philosopher Peter-Paul Verbeek (2005, p. 114), '[w]hat humans are and what their world is receive their form by artifactual mediation. Mediation does not simply take place *between* a subject and an object, but rather coshapes subjectivity and objectivity'. So, we should not think of technologies as neutral intermediaries interposed between humans and the physical world. Instead, we should see them as fully blown mediators affecting what it is to be in the world. Verbeek uses the example of a simple prosthesis: wearing glasses. When he wears his glasses, he is different. Glasses give him additional competencies and experiences. Without his glasses, some activities like writing are more difficult, while others like driving and piano playing are simply not possible.

Latour (1999) argues that technologies primarily permit mediation, in several senses. Technologies create interference. They create new programmes of action, new possibilities: you are a different person with a foot drop implant, gastric simulator, insulin pump or pacemaker. Technologies provide for new distributed practices, new compositions and new associations. They afford the exchange of performances and competencies. So, for example, a technology might do what a human once did. A doorperson can be replaced by an automatic door opener. Similarly, a technology might substitute for a human organ. A pacemaker does what a well-functioning heart would—specifically, what the electrical signals in the sinus or sinoatrial nodes would.

Third, non-humans are members of moral and political associations. We might think of this as morality materialised. We often get told to do things: drive slower, lose weight, stop smoking. These are inter-subjective commands; we may obey or not. To firm them up, they are often backed by political authority—the authority of the state, the force of the law. Thus, we get seat belt legislation, speeding tickets, smoking bans and other things such as driver education and smoking cessation programmes. Technologies enter too. Inter-subjective commands are woven in with inter-objective demands, and they become all the more compelling for it. Social norms and legal sanctions are strengthened by things. Computerised voices tell us off for not putting our seat belts on, beeps sound continuously, and the ignition refuses to work. The car is inoperable. Sensors encode morality. If I refuse to wear my seat belt, my car refuses to start. Dissent is not an option. Technologies perform regulatory roles. And not just in the realm of extrinsic politics—life 'out there'—but, thanks to PMDs, also in terms of intrinsic political roles, regulating life 'in here', too. They stabilise society, and they stabilise the self. Take, for instance, a news story of a woman who had endured years of incapacitating acid reflux. This made every meal a misery, disturbed her sleep and all but destroyed her social life. As part of a global trial, she was implanted with a device whose electric pulses stimulate the muscle valve at the base of the oesophagus, preventing or minimising reflux. Following the operation, food is now approached with pleasure rather than dread, and sleep is unproblematic. The newspaper headline ran: 'Implant Gives Reflux Sufferer Her Life Back' (Morton 2014).

Fourth, non-humans should be seen as gatherings. The limits of non-human agency should also be noted. Technologies do not have purpose and will and a sense of justice precisely as humans do, but they do still play a significant role in human associations. Non-humans gather actors from other times and places in a structured network. One of the implications here is that actors can act—which is to say, exert influence—when not present. Technologies extend us, which is one of the reasons for theorising them as prosthetics. Another point to reiterate is that any single thing only acts because of the other non-humans and humans that are associated with it. This was our point regarding socio-technical systems.

Latour (2002a, p. 249) uses the simple example of a hammer as a way of thinking about how technologies fold time and space. On the issue of time, the minerals in its composition are as old as the world itself, the wood in the handle will be of a significantly lesser age, and the time since it left the factory is less still. Latour's hammer holds together a German forest (the raw material for the shaft), a German mine (the raw material for the head), a German factory (the site of the hammer's production) and a French work van (the place of its sale). I would add something which Latour overlooks: the factory also folds in relation to production. Technologies delegate. They cross boundaries between symbols and things, and importantly they do the work that humans would otherwise have to do (and in the case of some PMDs like pacemakers, work that we can no longer do).

Technology, Life Itself and Life as Such

I have argued that individuals and individual technologies can be seen as network effects, enacted (or performed) by their socio-technical relations. This is a call for theorists to see the big picture, a point made in the preceding three sections. This section continues the theme by looking at the technology/politics/morality nexus today. In other words, I historicise the discussion by pausing to consider the contemporary human condition.

There has been a long-standing humanist tradition in which the actions (or consequences) of technology are greatly feared, the typical argument being that emerging technologies, whatever they may be, diminish our humanity. The fundamental question of what it is to be human underpins much of this. One of the most enduring motifs within technological theorising, and one of the longest voiced concerns, is that modern technologies are essentially dehumanising. This can be found in the work of Karl Marx on the rise of the objective machines of industrial modernity. Suddenly, the worker was reduced to a cog in the industrial apparatus, rather than being its controller. Equally, it can be found in some current theorising on the 'inner net' of the sensor society which we address in the section after next (Andrejevich and Burdon 2014; Turkle 2011).

PMDs are equally open to fears that we have somehow ceded agency, that we are no longer in control. Here, other concerns can be added that they threaten to extend life beyond natural life, whatever 'natural' life may be, or that they will extend humans beyond humans. Technological advances often lead to anxieties that we are going into a realm in which we do not properly belong, with consequent moral and ethical costs. Here, we can also note the costs accruing from the current political and demographic landscape, for in an age of austerity and with an ageing population, we are also talking about significant financial costs too. Interestingly, they are often advocated by those seeking to make savings (West 2013).

It may be helpful to note at this point that there is nothing new about arguments that technological advance is transgressing our humanity. Indeed, we have always used technology prosthetically, to go beyond ourselves, to surpass our physical limits. It is worth stressing that *this is one of the very points of technology*. As a species, we continue to extend our forces and, as Marshall McLuhan (2005, pp. 48–49) noted, since the electronic age, our senses as well.

Nigel Thrift (2005, p. 155) argues that throughout our history, there have been three great extensions of humans: the first was through writing, the second through machines (hardware) and the third through software. A number of PMDs are very much part of this third great extension (although they rely on the other two). And it is worth remembering that while they provide the prospect of new or prolonged ways of being in the world, they are very much part of an old debate.

As a counter to those arguments asserting technological degradation, a case can be made for technology as that which makes us human. Philosopher Bernard Stiegler (1998) argues that ours is a life form like no other, unique in that we are not simply life itself, but life always supported by, and dependent upon, technics. Stiegler uses 'technics' to denote the artificial, the inorganic, the technological, and through what they enable, the horizon of what is possible. We can think about this by going back to technology's very origins.

The oldest known technological object is a stone tool, found in the Olduvai Gorge in the East African Rift Valley, Tanzania (estimated age 1.8–2 million years old). The archaeological record shows that we have been using tools ever since. In fact, some suggest that we have been using tools for significantly longer, perhaps as long as 3.4 million years, which would mean that tool use precedes our own genus (Wong 2010). From the point of simplest tool use onwards, our evolution ceased to be merely genetic. It incorporated a 'new system of inheritance based not on the transmission of genes but of technical artefacts' (Stiegler 2011). Conceiving, creating and utilising technological objects have played a pivotal role in the development of our humanity: our history is entangled with technology. Some other animals use rudimentary objects, but no species other than the human species has constructed a complex socio-technical system. And in terms of object use, only humans manufacture them before they need them, exhibit an endless desire to improve them, anticipate their effects before they apply them and retain them for future use. Technology, then, is the difference that makes the difference: 'From the point where our ancestors started making tools … people have been unable to survive without the things they make; in this sense, it is making things that makes us human' (MacGregor 2010, p. 13).

There is, of course, a world of difference between the Stone Age society and contemporary existence, and as such Stiegler's philosophical abstractions on technology and humanity should be anchored in history and politics. Here, the suggestion is to locate discussions of PMDs and technology more broadly within the regimes that Nikolas Rose (2001) referred to as 'life itself' and to what Didier Fassin (2009) called 'life as such'.

Political authorities in Western societies have been deeply interested in the health and well-being of the population as a whole for the best part of a century and a half, as marked by the rise of the human and life sciences and clinical medicine, and the range of administrative practices from accident prevention all the way to town planning. In the academic literature, this has been most famously captured by Michel Foucault's (2010) scholarship on governmentality, which at once speaks to the art of government, the production of ideal populations, and the modes by which they are rendered governable. This is often described by another Foucauldian term: biopolitics (for an extended meditation on this see Lemke 2011).

This tracking of morbidity and mortality and targeted interventions to reduce their aggregate levels gave rise to a 'vital' politics (Rose 2001, p. 7). (I discuss vital technologies in the next section.) The older eugenic models based on notions of the defective have been displaced today by actuarial models based on risk. The growing salience of biotech and Big Pharma also means that interventions take place at the molecular level. Contemporary notions of selfhood also figure here: sociologists argue that the modern self is a project to be endlessly worked upon (Lawler 2014; Rose 2001, p. 18). To this, we must add the power of advertising in today's so-called consumer society, and the general ethos of neoliberalism whose politics have dominated for decades in most Western societies. Both exhort individuals to seek solutions to their problems through market mechanisms: we should buy the answers to our problems. Thus, we take pills to replace hormones, but we also take them to improve our fitness, lift our mood and enhance our sex drive.

From this, Rose concludes that what is significant about 'life itself' in our own times is the collapsing distinction between two things: (i) treatment and enhancement, and (ii) the natural and the prosthetic (which is where PMDs figure). He adds that management and enhancement of life is not simply the responsibility of the individual, but of their doctors *as well as* scientists, entrepreneurs and companies 'who make the reworking of life the object of their knowledge, inventions and products. Natural life can no longer serve as the ground or norm against which a politics of life may be judged' (Rose 2001, p. 17).

I reserve some scepticism towards the notion of 'natural life': what is it and when was it? But Rose's point that biomedical advances are giving us a range of choices that we never had before seems incontestable. With this in mind, it seems fruitful to refer to Didier Fassin's (2009) alternative anthropology of life, which he calls 'life as such'. This seems particularly apt given our knowledge of the social determinants of heath and given the hitherto unprecedented health disparities within Western nations, as well as between West and rest. Fassin (2009, p. 48) draws our attention 'to life as the course of events which occurs from birth to death, which can be shortened by political or structural violence, which can be prolonged by health or social policies, which gives place to cultural interpretations and moral decisions, which may be told or written—life which is lived through a body (not only through cells) and as a society (not only as a species)'.

It strikes me as being important to think through PMDs as embodied experience, and in relation to the connections between self and society, as well as in terms of human dignity: who deserves these technologies, who decides who can have them, and what level of care is received? As Fassin (2009, p. 57) writes, 'What politics does to life—and lives—is not just a question of discourses and technologies, of strategies and tactics. It is also a question of the concrete way in which individuals and groups are treated, under which principles and in the name of which morals, implying which inequalities and misrecognitions'.

New Technologies, New Distributions, New Challenges

In this section, I look at how PMDs act, giving particular emphasis to the ways that new PMDs can change scales, social forces, relations and conditions. I begin with the work of Marshall McLuhan. McLuhan (2005, p. 57) was well aware of the notion of technological agency and the consequences of technological adoption. He claimed that each new technological innovation creates its own environment. In follow-up work with son Eric, McLuhan identified a tetrad of scientific laws that they claimed applied to any media, indeed any technology. McLuhan and McLuhan (1988, p. 7) argue that we interrogate our technologies by asking of them: what do they intensify? What do they displace? What do they recapture? And what eventuates when they are pushed to extremes?

Their thinking can be applied to PMDs. Here, I reflect on debates regarding cochlear implants. In a strict biomedical sense, deafness may be seen as a disability, whereas for many insiders within the deaf community it is simply another way of being. Deafness is its own culture with its own mode of communication (particularly sign language). Seen thus, we are dealing with difference, not disability. And from this perspective, cochlear implants, when pushed to extremes (i.e. widespread mandatory use), would result in the destruction of deaf culture as it is currently practised. This would be nothing short of an act of cultural genocide. Recalling Fassin's points in the previous section, vital politics could here be read as a form of structural violence. Just because a technology allows us to do something, it does not follow that we should do it. There are important ethical questions to be addressed. *Can* does not imply *ought*.

We might also think about the McLuhans' points about changed relations and displacement. Amongst other things, the Internet allows for new modes of provision and procurement for medical technologies. This may downgrade, bypass or depersonalise the role of traditional medical authorities. The distribution channels for hearing aids are a case in point. Previously, they had gone through audiologists and other hearing specialists. Increasingly, insurers, pharmacies and large retailers like Wal-mart have moved into this domain. And now they are available through the Internet direct from manufacturers like America Hears and online retailers like Amazon. The technologies now self-program, although remote assistance is available.

Relatedly, the rise of peer-to-peer health care can be noted. According to the findings of the Pew Research Centre's Internet and American Life Project, over a third of all American adults have gone online to figure out a medical problem. From that group, 46% then went on to seek the advice of a medical professional, while 38% concluded that such actions were unnecessary. The Pew Research suggests that we are witnessing the rise of 'online diagnosers', who follow a certain pattern: they are more likely to be female than male, young than old, college-educated than not, and white rather than from an ethnic minority (Fox and Duggan 2013).

What this trend actually means is harder to say. The study cannot tell us if this trend is positive, negative or neutral, or for whom. They also remind readers that people have always reflected on the need for medical consultation, and it is only after a period of deliberation that most people go on to do so. (They can tell us that 70% of US adults sought information, care or support from a doctor or other health-care professional when a serious health issue presented.) Perhaps, then, the Internet merely adds another element to this process. It may even be considered a PMD in its own right. Perhaps, the Internet does just that, says Christine Moyer (2012) in a post on *American Medical News*, but physicians often argue that reading medical information online results in misdiagnosis and raised levels of anxiety. Plus, there is one diagnosis that patients are sure to miss: 'cyberchondria'.

There is one final point to be made about the potential of PMDs to redistribute relations. There are occasions when PMDs work too well, e.g.

when they are seen to prolong life-beyond-life. In such cases, complex ethical issues are brought up. Phillipa Malpas and Lisa Cooper (2012) discuss a New Zealand case in which a 75-year-old pacing-dependent woman was brought to the accident and emergency department of a public hospital. She had a brain injury and was in a coma, and it was thought that she would remain so until death by organ failure. The family requested that her pacemaker be deactivated. After some deliberations, the senior cardiac physiologist then reprogrammed the pacemaker to non-functioning mode. (will we see a growing role for technicians in this area?). The patient died shortly thereafter. The decision was made by assessing the clinical reality of her situation, her likely prognosis, the wishes of her husband and immediate family, and also their opinions of what they thought the patient would have wanted had they been able to articulate their own wishes. There was also a consultation with the hospital's legal team.

There have been suggestions in the literature that this constitutes a form of euthanasia. Expert bodies deny this. But it does seem that pacemakers may constitute a special case in the world of PMDs. L.A. Jansen (2006) makes precisely this argument, for three reasons: (1) spatial location—they are part of us, literally under our skin; (2) temporal duration—how long they have been part of us; and (3) they are life-sustaining. As Malpas and Cooper (2012) write, 'they are viewed as being part of the person's self'. On their view, stopping a pacemaker can be likened to hastening death by interfering with a patient's heart.

Technologies and Unintended Consequences: Lifehacking in the Sensor Society

This final section of my discussion thinks further through the social implications of these new technologies, their forms of monitoring and the technological systems that sustain them. It offers comment on subjectivity, social research, system abuse through surveillance and hacking, and (recalling our earlier points about thinking beyond the thing itself to consider supporting socio-technical systems) infrastructural provision.

Health apps and wearable technologies sell in their millions and make billions. Market research firm Markets and Markets (2015) produced a study predicting the mHealth market—which consists of connected devices, apps and monitoring services—to be worth almost $60 billion by 2020. (By comparison, it was worth just over $14 billion in 2015.) They highlight a number of related factors to account for this spectacular growth. In particular, they signal the growing number of smart devices, the enhanced use of connected medical devices and mHealth apps in health-care management (chronic diseases in particular), the increasing costs of health care (which incentivises cheaper treatment possibilities), the growing penetration of 3G and 4G networks and greater emphasis on patient-centred health-care provision.

Currently, the general health-care and fitness apps sector dominates the market. These PMDs offer new ways of knowing thyself, particularly the lifestyle ones which are sold (and bought) on the promise of empowerment (see Fitbit 2016). But what one has no way of knowing is the security of one's personal data, what 'normality' one is being measured against, the populations from which this benchmark data is derived, or the social assumptions that are built into the software's algorithms. Thinking back to our earlier point about the morality of technology, when we look at what gets built into health-monitoring technologies, we frequently find that the assumed user is a fit, white, middle-class male in the Global North (Lupton 2016). This, of course, assumes access, and access assumes both the necessary infrastructure to support it (e.g. Internet provision) and the ability to afford it as well as the apps and devices it enables. PMDs are therefore likely to open up yet another frontier of the digital divide, and be yet another means by which inequalities manifest.

Self-monitoring for health purposes is by no means new (Crawford et al. 2015), but M. Andrejevic and M. Burdon (2014) suggest that two connected trends most certainly are, and together they are transforming the worlds of information processing and surveillance. One is the proliferation of sensor technologies, those interactive networked devices that record and relay information, and the other is the rise of Big Data. An IBM (2013) report claims that 90% of the planet's stored data was created in the last 10 years.

When Sherry Turkle (2006) talked about 'the tethered self', it was largely in terms of our attachment to mobile devices. They are always on and always on us (and increasingly inside us). To which an important component must be added: they are always monitoring us too. This also creates new ways of being known. If technologies are implicated in the construction of society, we might reasonably ask what sort of world these technologies are helping to establish. For Andrejevic and Burdon (2014), ubiquitous media technologies and growing modes of data capture are contributing to the emergence of a new 'sensor society'.

Whereas the surveillance of old was discrete, targeted and purposeful (we may even say exceptional), the new sensor society continuously accumulates information: *It's the rule*. Data-mining displaces searching, patterns replace people. But this new logic of computation is somewhat opaque. The purposes for which information will be used, how it will be analysed and what will be discovered are all unclear, at least to individual users.

That there are powerful discoveries to be made is clear. Alex Pentland of the Massachusetts Institute of Technology tracked 60 families living in campus quarters using sensors and software in their smartphones. Records were made of movements, meetings, moods, physical health, social and spending habits. One of the claims made by this study is that '[b]y analyzing changes in movement and communication patterns, researchers could … detect flu symptoms before the students themselves realized they were getting sick'. Pentland stated: '[p]hones can know… People can get this god's-eye view of human behaviour' (cited in Hotz 2011).

This gives pause for thought about Big Data. It creates exciting new possibilities, but it also brings new risks. Pentland et al.'s study raises the unnerving possibility that others can come to know us better than we know ourselves. For this reason, many commentators suggest that the rise of these new monitoring technologies is creating the 'inner net' as technologies enter us and render more aspects of our being transparent. It has been a fundamental axiom of social science research that subjects are expert in their own lives. Implicit within Andrejevic and Burdon's (2014) piece is the suggestion that researchers will be less interested in soliciting subject beliefs. In preference, we will track behaviours.

Positivism 2.0 will follow a new logic of computation and find truth in the numbers. Andrejevic and Burdon signal alarm at the new and powerful forms of surveillance, the God's-eye view that the sensor society can give rise to. Who is watching? Why? What powerful new forms of information are they in possession of? They also worry about privacy issues: patterns, signals and digital traces can all be tracked back to individuals.

Marc Goodman (2012) offers further points on the downside of the Big Data digital revolution in his article 'Dark Data', reminding us that no technology has ever been produced that has not been hacked. Here, the Sony Playstation hack serves as a worrying precedent: 'more than 100 million people had their accounts compromised and their passwords stolen. Never before in human history has it been possible for one person to rob 100 million people—but our interconnectedness and mass data storage now make this possible' (Goodman 2012, p. 76). We are very used to ideas of identity theft and online fraud. But with the increased, and increasingly intimate, knowledge that accrues about us in the senor society, it seems that we are exposing ourselves (or being exposed by others) in profoundly new ways. We can change a password easily enough, but not our gender, and certainly not our height or blood group. And we might think about all those traces of us that get stored in various (and never totally secure) databases. The traffic between data centres is growing at a faster rate than the traffic from and to end-users (Mills 2013, p. 20).

Ominously, Goodman suggests that we are really only seeing the beginnings of cybercrime. The explosion of medical monitoring technologies—smart bracelets, smart phone apps that measure such parameters as blood sugar levels or brain activity—is particularly concerning. What happens when these technologies get hacked? What also of the swathe of medical implants that transmit digital data: cochlear implants, diabetic pumps, pacemakers and defibrillators? Over 60,000 Americans have pacemakers connected to the Internet. (And globally there are something like 600,000 pacemakers implanted annually.) How would these device users feel about others illegally accessing that data? How would they feel about the risk of their pacemaker being turned off? The phrase 'life hacking' is now commonly heard. It refers to tips and techniques, short cut and tricks through which life is made more productive or efficient. But life can be hacked in more visceral ways. Indeed, PMDs such as insulin pumps, pacemakers and defibrillators have already been hacked (Robertson 2012; Holpuch 2013).

The discussion thus far has conveyed a sense of the frailties inherent in these complex interconnected socio-technical systems. The same issues present in the infrastructures that support them. Energy grids are complex, tightly coupled systems. They are not merely infrastructure; they merit being described as critical infrastructure. Critical infrastructures are large-scale human-built systems that supply continual services central to society's functioning. Disruptions to critical infrastructures have rippling effects, as they are dynamic and interdependent arrangements. Electricity powers, connects to and synchronises with other systems. Graham (2010, p. 5) argues that it is more apt to think of separate infrastructures as a complex single whole. Blackouts affect pumps, refrigeration, traffic lights, trains and cell phone towers. This has serious consequences for water, waste, food, transportation and communication systems. Modern social life is impossible to imagine without it. Consider how essential electrical power is for the proper functioning of many PMDs. Indeed, PMDs could open up a new front of 'vital' technologies. Scholarship on vital technologies grows from the idea that in contemporary society citizenship is simultaneously political and technical, that to be a fully functioning member of society we need access to what Lakoff and Collier (2010) call 'material systems of circulation' like water, electrical power and communication systems.

The continuing sophistication and prevalence of electrical appliances only serves to increase our dependence. Here, digitisation is a key factor. In the digital world, interruptions and disturbances less than 1 cycle (1/60th second) can have catastrophic effects. Servers and computers crash; life support machines become their opposite; intensive care operations are compromised, as indeed are all manner of automated machines and microprocessor-based devices (Galvin Electricity Initiative 2011).[1]

Conclusion: We have Always been Prosthetic

David Harvey (2014, p. 97) writes that we are at a new point in the history of technological evolution: our technologies are now becoming 'biological' and are acquiring the types of properties that we associate with living organisms. In the case of PMDs, many may also be performing a role normally carried out biologically, and helping organisms to live thereby. These technologies are smart technologies that interact with their environment, self-monitor and sometimes self-repair. Technology, then, is now occupying a strange new domain between what W. Bryan Arthur (2009, p. 200) calls 'metabolism and mechanism'.

But we have always had to rely on things beyond our organic selves in order to survive. We have never been a closed system. This was Stiegler's point: human life has also always been technological. Opening up ourselves to our own reality will hopefully open up the space to properly theorise PMDs. Careful considerations need to be given to them, and we need to ask of PMDs what we would of all other technologies: who gets to access them, who produces them and under what conditions, what issues arise regarding ownership and control, how are they used and abused, and, noting the toxicity of e-waste, how are they to be disposed of? What intended and unintended consequences present themselves?

Medical devices permit competency in the world. We employ them for their efficacy. So it goes with all other technologies. If we think about prostheses in the literal senses of the word, as additions, applications and attachments, would we not say that all technologies are prostheses? They extend our bodies, forces and senses. They mediate our being in the world. Nikolas Rose (2001, p. 16) in a discussion of the transformational properties of drugs noted how they change people and their abilities through linking bodies with chemical actors: 'The body of the diabetic has been prosthetic since the invention of insulin treatment: calculated chemical artificiality here has sought to replace the missing or damaged normativity of the bodies own vital processes'. But if we turn to Stiegler or McLuhan, we could say that *we have always been prosthetic*.

The most famous prosthetic in Graeco-Roman antiquity was Pelops' replacement shoulder, fashioned from ivory. This was mythical, but there are others which arguably were not. In *The Natural History,* Pliny discusses Marcus Sergius, who lost his right hand in battle and had a replacement fashioned from iron. This did not seem to diminish his performance; Pliny felt him unsurpassed in valour.

Two things appeal about this idea of technologies as prosthetics: (1) it can be traced back to the origins of Western civilisation itself, and (2) it places theorising about personal medical devices at the very heart of things. This seems like a good place to end.

Note

1. Elsewhere, I have undertaken work with a colleague predicting increasing numbers of blackouts due to growing uncertainties in supply and growing certainties in demand. Supply will become increasingly precarious because of peak oil, political instability, industry liberalisation and privatisation, the precariousness of energy delivery systems, infrastructural neglect, global warming and the shift to renewable energy resources. Demand will become stronger because of population growth, rising levels of affluence and the consumer 'addictions' which accompany it (Byrd and Matthewman 2014). Curiously, very little health research seems to have been done on the impacts of blackouts. The first literature review on it was produced by Public Health England (Klinger et al. 2014).

References

Andrejevic, M., & Burdon, M. (2014). Defining the sensor society. *Television and New Media.* doi:10.1177/1527476414541552.

Arthur, W. (2009). *The nature of technology: What it is and how it evolves.* London: Penguin.

Barad, K. (2003). Posthumanist performativity: Toward an understanding of how matter comes to matter. *Signs: Journal of Women in Culture and Society, 28*(3), 801–831.

Bijker, W. (2010). How is technology made?—That is the question! *Cambridge Journal of Economics, 34,* 63–76.

Byrd, H., & Matthewman, S. (2014). Exergy and the city: The technology and sociology of power (failure). *Journal of Urban Technology, 21*(3), 85–102.

Callon, M., & Latour, B. (1981). Unscrewing the big leviathan. In K. Knorr-Cetina & M. Mulkay (Eds.), *Advances in social theory and methodology* (pp. 275–303). London: Routledge and Kegan Paul.

Connor, S. (2008). Thinking things. In *Extended Version of a Plenary Lecture Given at the 9th Annual Conference of the European Society for the Study of English, Aarhus, Denmark, 25 August.* Available online at http://stevenconnor.com/thinkingthings.html. Accessed September 12, 2016.

Crawford, K., Lingel, J., & Karppi, T. (2015). Our metrics, ourselves: A hundred years of self-tracking from the weight scale to the wrist wearable device. *European Journal of Cultural Studies, 18*(4–5), 479–496.

Drucker, P. F. (2006). *Classic Drucker.* Cambridge, MA: Harvard Business School .

Fassin, D. (2009). Another politics of life is possible. *Theory, Culture & Society, 26*(5), 44–60.

Fitbit. (2016). *Who we are.* Available online at https://www.fitbit.com/nz/about. Accessed June 20, 2016.

Foucault, M. (2010). *The government of self and others: Lectures at the Collège de France 1982–1983.* Basingstoke: Palgrave Macmillan.

Fox, S., & Duggan, M. (2013). Health online 2013. *Pew Research Internet Project.* Available online at http://www.pewinternet.org/2013/01/15/health-online-2013/. Accessed January 8, 2014.

Galvin Electricity Initiative. (2011). *The electric power system is unreliable.* Available online at http://www.galvinpower.org/resources/library/fact-sheets-faqs/electric-power-system-unreliable. Accessed January 8, 2014.

Goodman, M. (2012). Dark data. In R. Smolan & J. Erwitt (Eds.), *The human face of big data* (pp. 74–77). Against All Odds Productions: Sausalito.

Graham, S. (Ed.). (2010). *Disrupted cities: When infrastructure fails.* New York: Routledge.

Harvey, D. (2014). *Seventeen contradictions and the end of capitalism.* London: Profile.

Holpuch, A. (2013, July 29). Hacker Barnaby Jack's cause of death could remain unknown for months. *The Guardian.* Available online at http://www.theguardian.com/technology/2013/jul/29/barnaby-jack-hacker-cause-of-death. Accessed August 28, 2013.

Hotz, R. (2011, April 23). What they know: The really smart phone. *The Wall Street Journal* . Available online at http://online.wsj.com/news/articles/SB1 0001424052748704547604576263261679848814. Accessed June 20, 2016.

IBM. (2013). *The IBM Big Data Platform.* IBM Software Group. Available online at http://public.dhe.ibm.com/common/ssi/ecm/en/imb14135usen/ IMB14135USEN.PDF. Accessed June 20, 2016.

Jansen, L. (2006). Hastening death and the boundaries of the self. *Bioethics, 20*(2), 105–111.

Khoo, M. (2005). Technologies aren't what they used to be: Problematising closure and relevant social groups. *Social Epistemology, 19*(3), 283–285.

Klinger, C., Landeg, O., & Murray, V. (2014, January 2) Power outages, extreme events and health: A systematic review of the literature from 2011–2012. *PLoS Currents 6.* Available online at http://www.ncbi.nlm.nih.gov/pmc/articles/PMC3879211/. Accessed June 18, 2016.

Lakoff, A., & Collier, S. (2010). Infrastructure and event: The political technology of preparedness. In B. Braun & S. Whatmore (Eds.), *Political matter: Technoscience, democracy and public life* (pp. 243–266). Minneapolis: University of Minnesota Press.

Latour, B. (1992). *Where are the missing masses? Sociology of a door.* Available online at http://www.bruno-latour.fr/sites/default/files/50-MISSING-MASSES-GB.pdf. Accessed September 12, 2016.

Latour, B. (1999). *Pandora's hope: Essays on the reality of science studies.* Cambridge, MA: Harvard University Press.

Latour, B. (2002a). Technology and morality: The ends of means. *Theory, Culture & Society, 19*(5–6), 247–260.

Latour, B. (2002b). There is no information, only transformation: An interview with Bruno Latour. In G. Lovink (Ed.), *Uncanny networks: Dialogues with the virtual intelligentsia* (pp. 154–160). Cambridge, MA: MIT Press.

Latour, B. (2005). *Reassembling the social: An introduction to Actor-Network theory*. Oxford: Oxford University Press.

Law, J. (1992). Notes on the theory of the Actor-Network: Ordering, strategy, and heterogeneity. *Systems Practice, 5*(4), 379–393.

Law, J., & Bijker, W. (Eds.). (1992). *Shaping technology/building society: Studies in sociotechnical change*. Cambridge, MA: MIT Press.

Lawler, S. (2014). *Identity: Sociological perspectives* (2nd ed.). Cambridge: Polity.

Lemke, T. (2011). *Bio-politics: An advanced introduction*. New York: New York University Press.

Lupton, D. (2013). Understanding the human machine [commentary]. *IEEE Technology and Society Magazine, 32*(4), 25–30.

Lupton, D. (2016). Digital risk society. *This Sociological Life*. Available online at https://simplysociology.wordpress.com/. Accessed June 20, 2016.

MacGregor, N. (2010). *A history of the world in 100 objects*. London: Allen Lane.

MacKenzie, D., & Wajcman, J. (Eds.). (1985). *The social shaping of technology*. Milton Keynes: Open University Press.

Malpas, P., & Cooper, L. (2012). The ethics of deactivating a pacemaker in a pacing-Dependent patient. Reflections on a case study. *American Journal of Hospice and Palliative Medicine, 29*(7), 566–569.

Markets and Markets. (2015). mHealth Solutions Market by Connected Devices (Blood Pressure Monitor, Glucose Meter, Pulse Oximeter) Apps (Weight Loss, Women's Health, Personal Health Record, & Medication) Services (Remote Monitoring, Consultation, Prevention)—Global Forecast to 2020. Available online at http://www.marketsandmarkets.com/PressReleases/mhealth-apps-and-solutions.asp. Accessed June 20, 2016.

Matthewman, S. (2011). *Technology and social theory*. Basingstoke: Palgrave Macmillan.

McLuhan, M. (2005). *Understanding me: Lectures and interviews*. Toronto: MIT Press.

McLuhan, E., & McLuhan, M. (1988). *Laws of media: The new science*. Toronto: University of Toronto Press.

Mills, M. (2013). *The cloud begins with coal: Big data, big networks, big infrastructure, and big power*. Digital Power Group. Available online atwww.techpundit.com/wp-content/uploads/2013/07/Cloud_Begins_With_Coal.pdf. Accessed June 18, 2016.

Morton, J. (2014),22 January. Implant gives reflux sufferer her life back. *The New Zealand Herald*.Available online at http://www.nzherald.co.nz/lifestyle/news/article.cfm?c_id=6&objectid=11310801. Accessed June 20, 2016.

Moyer, C. S. (2012), 30 January. Cyberchondria: The one diagnosis patients Miss. *American Medical News*. Available online at http://www.amednews.com/article/20120130/health/301309952/1/. Accessed August 25, 2014.

Pfaffenberger, B. (1992). Technological dramas. *Science, Technology and Human Values, 17*(3), 282–312.

Robertson, J. (2012, March 1). McAfee Hacker says Medtronic insulin pumps vulnerable to attack. *Bloomberg*. Available online athttp://www.bloomberg. com/news/2012-02-29/mcafee-hacker-says-medtronic-insulin-pumps-vulnerable-to-attack.html. Accessed August 28, 2013.

Rose, N. (2001). The politics of life itself. *Theory, Culture & Society, 18*(6), 1–30.

Rotman, B. (2008). *Becoming beside ourselves: The alphabet, ghosts, and distributed human being*. Durham, NC: Duke University Press.

Sayes, E. (2014). Actor-Network Theory and methodology: Just what does it mean to say that nonhumans have agency? *Social Studies of Science, 44*(1), 134–149.

Shah, S., & Robinson, I. (2008). Medical device technologies: Who is the user? *International Journal of Healthcare Technology and Management, 9*(2), 181–197.

Stiegler, B. (1998). *Technics and time: The fault of epimetheus*. Stanford: Stanford University Press.

Stiegler, B. (2011). This system does not produce pleasure anymore: An interview with Bernard Stiegler. *Krisis: Journal for Contemporary Philosophy 1*. Available online at http://krisis.eu/content/2011-1/krisis-2011-1-05-lemmens.pdf. Accessed June 20, 2016.

Thrift, N. (2005). *Knowing capitalism*. London: Sage.

Turkle, S. (2006). *Always-on / always-on-you*: The tethered self. Available online at http://web.mit.edu/sturkle/www/Always-on%20Always-on-you_The%20 Tethered%20Self_ST.pdf. Accessed May 27, 2010.

Turkle, S. (2011). *Alone together: Why we expect more from technology and less from each other*. New York: A.A. Knopf.

Verbeek, P. (2005). *What things do: Philosophical reflections on technology*. University Park: Pennsylvania State University Press.

West, D. (2013). *Improving healthcare through mobile medical devices and sensors*. Washington, DC: The Brookings Institution.

Winner, L. (1977). *Autonomous technology: Technics-out-of-control as a theme in political thought*. Cambridge, MA: MIT Press.

Winner, L. (1980). Do artifacts have politics? *Daedalus, 109*(1), 121–136.

Wong, K. (2010). Ancient cut marks reveal far earlier origin of Butchery. *Scientific American*. Available online athttp://www.scientificamerican.com/ article/ancient-cutmarks-reveal-butchery/. Accessed June 20, 2016.

Part II

Reconstructing the Personal: Bodies, Selves and Pmds

While PMDs are usually thought of in relation to their use by individuals, the realities of technology-in-use typically involve a wider range of relationships and networks. Moreover, though PMDs are often conceptualised as neutral pieces of technology clinically placed on otherwise unchanged bodies, technology usage can transform bodies and selves as well as monitoring and treating them. Consequently, this part of the book will explore various kinds of networks, bodies and selves created through PMDs in different contexts. Chapter 3 foregrounds the meaning-making work undertaken by individuals using PMDs (ovulation monitors and consumer gene tests) and engaging in online forums to make sense of their technological practices. This chapter shows how discussion and speculation, artefacts and bodily sensations, and anticipations and corporeal imaginaries are drawn together through shared experiences of PMDs in order to constitute the 'biosensing body.' Chapters 4 and 5 take a more micro-scale focus, drawing on ethnographic data to consider how bodies and selves are mediated and constructed through PMDs such as insulin pumps for people with type 1 diabetes (Chap. 4) and a range of wellness and fitness devices (Chap. 5). Across these different PMD use contexts, individual bodily boundaries are altered and extended through user–technology interaction, leading to new constructions of self and agency. Through these chapters, it becomes apparent that PMDs not only influence and create different understandings of health and experiences of healthcare, but also impact on our conceptualisations of who we are and what we can do.

3

Biosensing Networks: Sense-Making in Consumer Genomics and Ovulation Tracking

Mette Kragh-Furbo, Joann Wilkinson, Maggie Mort, Celia Roberts and Adrian Mackenzie

Introduction

What happens when personal medical devices in the form of health bio-sensors move out of clinical settings and control and into commercial and online environments? How do individual 'users'[1] make sense of the large

M. Kragh-Furbo (✉) · J. Wilkinson · M. Mort ·
C. Roberts · A. Mackenzie
University of Lancaster, Lancaster, UK
e-mail: m.kraghfurbo@lancaster.ac.uk

J. Wilkinson
e-mail: j.wilkinson@lancaster.ac.uk

M. Mort
e-mail: m.mort@lancaster.ac.uk

C. Roberts
e-mail: celia.roberts@lancaster.ac.uk

A. Mackenzie
e-mail: a.mackenzie@lancaster.ac.uk

© The Author(s) 2018
R. Lynch and C. Farrington (eds.), *Quantified Lives and Vital Data*,
Health, Technology and Society, https://doi.org/10.1057/978-1-349-95235-9_3

amounts of 'data' which arise from engagement with health biosensors? What do their sense-making practices tell us about sensing and knowing the body? In this chapter, we focus on two different kinds of biosensors: the gene test offered by the consumer genomics company 23andMe and a fertility monitor (the ovulation microscope). Both promise new insights into the body—insights that enable users to know the body in different ways. The companies that sell these devices claim that users will be able to get to know their genetic susceptibilities or identify when they ovulate. Yet, making sense of the genotype data and microscope images is not always as straightforward as advertised. We focus here on the practices by which users work their way to understandings of the biosensing body. We characterise this as a material-semiotic process involving a number of different actors and materials. Where health data is worked on in commercial, domestic and online domains rather than within clinically controlled settings, new actors and objects come into play, which start to shape knowledge of the body in various ways. Our analysis shows that knowledge of the body is therefore not simply 'found' in the devices.

Based on two ethnographic studies of online forums where individuals discuss and work on their biosensor data, we argue that individuals make sense of biosensor data by engaging in socio-material networks of biosensing. This is sense-making by doing, where individuals engage with each other online and together attempt to make sense of their bodies, specifically ovulation and genetic susceptibility. This involves discussion, speculation and imagination as well as the sharing of test results, documents and other online material. It also involves a kind of care that—often taking place alongside clinical care—operates through speculations and conversations with fellow forum participants as well as through material practice. This is not care as a product or service, but a kind of care that prioritises conversation and imagination. Although care is 'a slippery word' (Martin et al. 2015, p. 625), Maria Puig de la Bellacasa (2011, p. 100) argues that care is a kind of practice that is 'a vital necessity in our technoscientific world [...] [N]othing holds together in a liveable way without caring relationships'.

We draw on science and technology studies (STS) approaches to help theorise the body as made across a network of multiple and heterogeneous actors. The body and its stuff are not given, 'natural' objects discovered by science or medicine but, as Bruno Latour (2005) has argued, hybrid entities existing in and constituted by a network of forces and practices. In these 'actor-networks', there is heterogeneity, which means the presence of different actors, human and non-human, and there is semiotic relationality, which means that the different actors within the network define and shape one another (Law 2009). The networks are also 'material-semiotic', which means that nature and bodies are never outside language or discourse (Haraway 1997). Instead, bodies materialise within structures of power and knowledge that might involve institutions, narratives, technical practices, labour or legal structures, and much more. We also draw on Latour's suggestion (2004, pp. 206–207) that we talk about the body in terms of 'learning to be affected'. The body is understood to be 'a progressive enterprise that produces at once a sensory medium *and* a sensitive world'. This is essential, Latour argues, to a body's becoming and how we inhabit the world, and importantly, this capacity to be affected or moved into action is achieved through a collective body or what he calls 'artificial layered set-ups' that consist of humans, non-humans and hybrid forms. To theorise the body as emerging in material-semiotic practice thus means that we do not take the body for granted and that we bring both discourse and materials into the same analytical view. When we ask *how do individuals make sense of their biosensor data?* we pay attention to how this is done in material-semiotic practice and what participates in these processes. We can then say more about how the biosensing body is constituted and held together in 'actor-networks' and how individuals acquire (or learn to have) a biosensing body.

In the next section, we introduce the two biosensors through a discussion of the promises and claims made about them, such as control of the body through knowledge, albeit in different ways. We then analyse and discuss each biosensing practice. We report on findings from two ethnographic studies that have focused on consumer genomics (Kragh-Furbo) and ovulation monitoring (Wilkinson), respectively. The studies have been part of the project 'Living Data: Making Sense of Health Biosensors', carried out at Lancaster University, which also included a citizens' panel study (Mort et al. 2016). The project has been part of a broader interdisciplinary and international research programme—Biosensors in Everyday Life—supported by Intel's University Research Office (2010–2013) and led by anthropologist Dawn Nafus (2016).

Health Biosensors for Sale: Their Claims and Promises

Health biosensors are forms of personal medical devices that work with bodily material to say something about the body. They combine bodily fluids (e.g. saliva or urine) with a form of physiochemical detector to analyse the bodily substance and convert it into some kind of signal or pattern (Nafus 2016). Yet, what signals, patterns or numbers say about the body, for example ovulation or genetic susceptibilities, has to be worked out in practice. The two kinds of health biosensors studied are both taken up in a response to significant life changes—pregnancy and illness—both of which are constituted by new modes of acquiring health data as well as (to some extent) similar sense-making practices. They are both available to purchase direct-to-consumer. 23andMe's Personal Genome Service can be purchased via their website or in-store in the UK for £125 ($199 in the USA). The ovulation microscopes are also sold online and in-store, priced at approximately £20. The 23andMe gene test works by the user spitting into a vial and shipping the sample to 23andMe's contracted laboratory that analyses the customer's DNA to provide her/him with genetic reports on inherited conditions, disease risks, drug response, traits and ancestry. The ovulation microscope, on the other hand, encourages women to repeatedly test for the changes in hormone levels in their saliva over a specific period of time. The ovulation monitor, in the context of trying to conceive, is thus purpose specific and time limited, while the consumer gene test presents an endless array of health-related practices. While the two kinds of health biosensors involve contrasting temporalities as well as different purposes and aims, by considering the two together we are able to draw attention to the practices and doings that are woven into multiple sense-making contexts and spaces.

While some biosensors, e.g. the pregnancy test, have been on the market for many years, recent developments in science and technology have enabled newly networked forms of measuring and profiling. Such new devices, Nick Fox (2015, p. 13) comments, 'are of profound sociological interest because they manifest affect economies that reflect a range of inter-connected technical, medical, personal and business affectivities and associated micropolitical engagements'. Fox notes how the blood pressure monitor, for example, assembles relations between the vascular system, device, user, manufacturer, biomedicine and health professionals, in which the user, in this assemblage, is made responsible for both monitoring and action in response to the readings. The biomedical gaze thus extends into domestic spaces, and medical monitoring is outsourced and privatised. Bodies are increasingly drawn into biomedical jurisdiction (Clarke et al. 2003, p. 162) in which the management of health and illness is considered in terms of 'individual moral responsibilities to be fulfilled through improved access to knowledge, self-surveillance, prevention, risk assessment, the treatment of risk, and the consumption of appropriate self-help/biomedical goods and services'.

Many of the new health biosensors also see data flows between devices, consumers, companies, institutions, social networks and back again, and in many cases, the user never sees how the data is analysed, sold or repurposed (Crawford et al. 2015). While the domestic weight scale, for example, and new health biosensors both offer the promise of agency through mediated self-knowledge, Crawford et al. (2015, p. 495) note how the new devices come with 'a range of capital-driven imperatives and standard-making exercises that seek to normalize and extract value from our understanding of ourselves, while making us ever more knowable to an emerging set of data-driven interests'. Health biosensors are argued to add a new layer of surveillance, which then brings about questions of control, access and the interpretation of personal biosensing data (Crawford et al. 2015; see also Lupton 2014). For example, arguments have been made for the work involved in health biosensors as free labour (e.g. Till 2014; Harris et al. 2013). In their study of the consumer genomics company 23andMe's research practices, Anna Harris, Sally Wyatt and Susan E. Kelly (Harris et al. 2013) have argued that while 23andMe presents its research participation as a form of gift exchange, the gift is used to draw attention away from the free, clinical labour undertaken by its customers. When people purchase 23andMe's Personal Genome Service, they are also invited to participate in the company's genetics research by donating their DNA to research as well by filling out online questionnaires about their health and illness. This free clinical labour, Harris et al. argue, is what drives the profitability of 23andMe. Yet this is not made clear to customers.

What is sold, however, is often a promise 'to enhance the legibility of bodily signs', as Ana Viseu and Lucy Suchman (2010, p. 163) put it—that is, to make unknown or invisible aspects of the body detectable and transparent. This is meant to encourage 'an associated responsibility to act, and more specifically to act within intensified regimes of self improvement and bodily control' (ibid). In the case of 23andMe's Personal Genome Service, it promises 'a new kind of knowledge' that enables 'you to make more informed choices about your diet and exercise', lets you 'explore what makes you unique' and allows you to encounter 'a new way to see yourself' (23andMe.com 2015). These discourses reflect what Carlos Novas and Nikolas Rose (2000) have called 'the birth of the somatic individual', and they map onto Rose's (2007, p. 8) suggestion that 'we are seeing the emergence of a novel somatic ethics, imposing obligations yet imbued with hope, oriented to the future yet demanding action in the present.' At least, that is what is imagined.

Yet, and this is our concern, test results are not always immediately useful or actionable. Interpreting genetic susceptibilities or ovulation microscope images can be difficult. Using these devices, it is often assumed that the data will make sense to the user. However, as we go on to show, this is not always the case. To some extent, 23andMe acknowledges that more interpretative work is needed. While the company does not provide genetic counselling as part of its service, 23andMe does encourage its customers to contact a healthcare professional, providing links to genetic counselling services on its website. Therefore, while 23andMe attempts to disrupt traditional medical power relations through a so-called democratisation of access to information (Fiore-Gartland and Neff 2016) in offering its Personal Genome Service direct-to-consumer, the company still relies on parts of the medical system. 'Disruption discourses [also] ignore the fact that data require mediation' (Fiore-Gartland and Neff 2016, p. 119)—i.e. interpretative work done by medical professionals or by individuals themselves.

Health biosensors also introduce questions about how we come to know the body, and ultimately, the relationship between sensing, seeing and knowing bodies. In this way, the focus shifts from 'what is ovulation or genetic susceptibility?' to 'how do we come to know these?' The relationship between knowing and sensing has been addressed by Barbara Duden (1993) in her study of the diaries of an eighteenth-century German doctor. Duden (1993, p. 141) observes a very different framework for understanding the realities of the body, in which 'illness-causing phenomena was conceived as part of a logic of the life story, not as part of the logic of the body as such'. Illness and the body were understood through everyday life events and physical sensations and not through descriptions of organs, systems or body parts. Valerie Hartouni (1997, p. 12) adds to this discussion through an exploration of 'seeing' as a learned event: 'Seeing is a set of learned practices that allow us to organise the visual field and that engage us in producing the world that we seem to greet and take in only passively'. Technologies such as ultrasound and fibre-optic imagining, she adds, are peering technologies, but they do not simply 'turn the inside out, render the oblique transparent or extend our vision to reveal the elusive secrets of nature. Technologies themselves do not peer; they are *instruments* and *relations* that facilitate or obstruct but, above all, construct "peering"' (Hartouni 1997, p. 64). Hartouni thus criticises the notion of a reality 'out there' which later comes to represent a truth. For her, there is no neutral or passive vision, but only ever a vision which has been organised and coded. Bernike Pasveer (1989), in her study of the introduction of X-rays into medicine, also shows how 'the knowledge of shadows' is shaped by the activities of X-ray workers, as they experiment with the technology and the images in practice. Learning from these studies, we discuss not what ovulation microsopes or gene tests show, but how individuals make sense of them through discussion, speculation and collaboration as well as material practice.

Researching Biosensor Networks

We have observed and collected data from a number of online forums where people discuss and interpret their biosensor data. There are thousands of online forums today and many are health oriented, e.g. the large patient network PatientsLikeMe (www.patientslikeme.com). We have observed a subsection of a large online forum for people living with a chronic illness, which we here call SNPnet. We have also observed the 'trying to conceive' subsections of four different online parenting forums, which we will refer to as the 'Fertility Forums'. We observed the forums over a period of 12 months where data was collected and subsequently analysed. Prior to the start of the research, permission to observe and collect data was sought and granted from forum administrators. We have used pseudonyms to protect the identity of the forum and its participants, although we acknowledge that full protection is impossible given the public nature of the forums.[2]

It is important to reflect here on the particularities of online data and what this may offer for researchers within the social sciences. For Christine Hine (2008), online exchanges should not be viewed as interactions but instead as a collection of 'texts' which produce different kinds of interpretive encounters from face-to-face communication. One area of tension within textual practices relates to the authenticity of the users in terms of their 'real identities'; issues arise as to whether online/offline lives correspond, and if users *really are* what they write. In this sense, offline worlds become a standard to which online worlds are compared, as Hine notes: '[f]ace to face interaction is often taken as a "gold standard" for rich and truthful interaction, despite all our experiences to the contrary' (Hine 2008, p. 264). Research online therefore allows for a reflection on what it means to be authentic and authenticity's putative link with embodiment (Markam 2003). Along similar lines, the work of Richard Rogers (2013) on digital methods aims to deflect interest away from the seemingly real/unreal divide of the internet towards a notion of this as an object of study and as an important source for understanding cultural change and societal conditions. Rogers (2013, p. 19) makes an ontological distinction between 'objects' that are born online (natively digital) and ones that have migrated there (digitised), thus rechannelling the way in which findings from studies of online worlds are 'grounded' or calibrated with offline contexts.

The Online Forums

SNPnet is part of a non-profit organisation that provides online support for people living with a particular chronic illness. The organisation maintains an online forum with several sub-forums, for example, on events, news and research, symptoms, diagnosis and treatment, and so forth. For the purpose of this chapter, we focus on the sub-forum that we call SNPnet, where members discuss genetic mutations (or single nucleotide polymorphisms or SNPs—hence the name of the sub-forum) and treatment protocols. The sub-forum has a small number of active participants who regularly post and comment; many of these participants have been ill for some time. The site also has a larger group of participants, who appear now and again on the feeds, but who do not tend to engage in detailed discussions about SNPs. Like other forums, the sub-forum has an unknown number of 'lurkers', who only rarely post or comment on forum threads, or not at all.

Members of SNPnet discuss their results from consumer gene tests and attempt to connect these to knowledge of metabolism and supplementation in order to begin or improve treatment protocols that focus on diet and health supplementation. It is suggested that with the right supplementation, it is possible to improve the metabolism of certain chemicals in the body and thus help to relieve some of their illness symptoms. This is based on the theories of methylation and nutrigenomics, which have been taken up by a number of alternative medical practitioners[3]—most notably Amy Yasko (www.dramyyasko.com) and Ben Lynch (www.mthfr.net). In her book 'Pathways to Recovery', Amy Yasko describes methylation deficiencies as the under- or over-activation of methylation, which is 'a key cellular pathway that promotes detoxification, controls inflammation, and balances the neurotransmitters [and] can result in mood and emotional shifts as well as liver, pancreas, stomach, intestinal, adrenal, thyroid, and hormonal imbalances'

(Yasko 2004, p. 15). Treatment protocols have been suggested to help optimise these methylation deficiencies and restore methylation function, and with the help of genetic testing, it is suggested that it is possible to target these biochemical imbalances with 'the missing nutritional ingredients that the body cannot adequately produce itself due to genetic mutations' (ibid, p. 23). While Yasko focuses on children with autism, she also treats a number of other chronic illnesses applying the same knowledge and protocols. A simplified version of Yasko's treatment protocol has been posted on SNPnet, and many of the sub-forum participants try to work out their own treatment protocols with the help from her website and books. Yasko does not contribute to the discussions on SNPnet.

The 'Fertility Forums' are situated within larger online parenting forums which provide support and advice on a range of topics, often family related, but sometimes on work or everyday life issues. All the forums house a specific subsection dealing with fertility and conception. These are frequently divided into multiple areas of interest such as 'waiting to try', 'not trying, not preventing', 'long-term trying to conceive' and 'secondary infertility'. The women who write on the forums vary in age from early twenties to mid- or late forties, and although few details regarding professional lives are given, most of the women refer to their employment at some point when posting. The frequency of posts varies also, with some writing weekly, daily or several times on one day if the thread in question is of interest to them.

Women use the forums for support or advice on conception, or for information on health supplements which may affect the ovulation cycle or cervical mucous. Many discussions on the forums also centre on specific biosensing devices and practices, and how to understand the data that is collected. The 'Fertility Forums' display posts from women who are just beginning to unravel conception in terms of ovulation, eggs, sperm and cervical mucous as well as from those who have come to be considered—sometimes by themselves, often by others—as knowledgeable or as (lay) 'experts'. In some posts, women who are regular contributors to the forum will make references to more knowledgeable members of the group. However, greater fertility knowledge is viewed, in part, as an unfortunate indication that a woman has been trying to conceive for a long time, and is potentially infertile. It is important to add nonetheless that women who write in these sections range from identifying as 'beginning to try to conceive' to 'experiencing difficulty' in trying to conceive, but never as 'infertile' or unable to have children.

SNPnet and the 'Fertility Forums' are spaces where individuals can discuss with others, share their experiences and ask questions of each other, and spaces through which biosensor data is reconfigured as it moves across and in between hardware, interfaces and people's lives. As we show, the sub-forums become spaces for collaboration where participants work together in a wide range of ways to make sense of their data and bodies. This work involves discussions and negotiations over test results and how to use the devices, as well as conversations based on speculation, hypothesis and personal experiences.

Making Sense of Genetic Susceptibilities

On SNPnet, many open questions are asked, such as 'what do I need to know?' and 'how do I get started on this?' For many of the participants, it is not obvious how their genetic data is useful or actionable. Together, however, they come to work this out—at least partially. Yet, it is often presumed that the data is useful, and that it is simply a matter of working out how it is useful. This sense of potential as well as hope is partially a result of how others on the forum claim to have improved their symptoms by incorporating this data into their treatment protocols. However, it must also be understood in relation to the multi-layered problematisation that accompanies the nature of a contested chronic illness and the lives of people with this illness. While some sub-forum participants also receive support from medical professionals, others do not. Instead, they find support online.[4] On SNPnet, they become participants who contribute to discussions about genetic susceptibilities and supplementation. This is different from becoming members of a formal patient organisation or health activist group. Many patient organisations, in addition to helping patients manage their illness, also actively intervene in a 'war on disease', e.g. by getting involved in research and clinical efforts to fight the disease (Rabeharisoa et al. 2014). Patients may become 'lay experts' in that they acquire scientific and medical knowledge and become 'genuine participants in the process of knowledge construction' (Epstein 1995, p. 409). While SNPnet is part of an organisation that provides information to support people with a certain chronic illness, the sub-forum is not a patient organisation in this sense.

Nonetheless, the sub-forum's participants become knowledgeable in a different way as they learn to have a biosensing body through the sense-making work that happens on and through the forum. This resembles what Jeanette Pols (2014, p. 75) calls 'practical *knowing in action*', which is also 'daily practices of knowing rather than […] a body of knowledge'. It is a kind of knowledge that is equivalent, Pols argues, to clinical knowledge, but rather than 'coaching or treating different individual patients… patients use and develop this practical knowledge to translate knowledge from different sources … into usable techniques, and coordinate this with the different aims they have in life, in a context that is always changing' (Pols 2014, p. 78).

The sense-making work taking place on SNPnet involves sharing of genetic data and personal biographies, discussions of online texts and reading materials, the use of DIY-style analysis tools, and making suggestions for health supplements and diet based on what they read and learn from others. The participants juggle complex medical knowledge and scientific research and how this knowledge maps (or not) on to their own genetic data and personal experiences. They read about and discuss genetic mutations, methylation, gene expression and other genetic concepts and processes. Drawing on a number of online resources (most often websites such as heartfixer.com, Wikipedia and SNPedia, but also PubMed, dbSNP and OMIN), participants will try to piece together some kind of answer, although well aware that what they piece together will necessarily be partial. In the extract below, a participant asks about the significance of the MAO-A enzyme and how to interpret the test results (genotypes).

This is the wikipedia article on MAO-A: http://en.wikipedia.org/wiki/Monoamine_oxidase_A

It talks about inhibitors at the bottom, but I don't yet understand, does a T mean that I have LOW or HIGH levels of the related MAO-A enzyme?

Looking at the heartfixer site, it seems to be saying that the enzyme that this gene expresses is supposed to turn serotonin into HIAA, which I think is this stuff:

http://en.wikipedia.org/wiki/5-Hydroxyindoleacetic_acid

[…] Well, I welcome anyone's thoughts or knowledge on this.

Janine, SNPnet, posted 27 March 27 2012.

Others join the discussion and more links are shared. They share what they know about the MAO-A enzyme, and what the genotype T might mean in relation to the breakdown of serotonin in the body. They draw on their own experiences and what they have read online, for example, from Yasko's work. They speculate and try to come up with some answers. Yet, those are constantly tweaked as others join in and add to the discussions with more links, their data analysis reports and personal experiences. As the discussion continues, the uncertainty that surrounds this kind of sense-making becomes more evident, but nonetheless, something that is managed, to some extent, through discussions and sharing with others.[5]

While uncertainty necessarily accompanies this data practice, there is also an excitement about the unknown: 'The thing is that we are kind of pioneers here. It's a brave new and mostly unexplored world' (SNPnet, posted 27 March 2012). In genomics research as well as consumer genomics, there is scope for irrelevant data, and to some extent, this is also evident on the sub-forum. While the sub-forum participants tend to focus on a dozen or so SNPs in their negotiations and analyses, which SNPs are relevant to their treatment protocols have not been agreed on either by the scientific or by the medical community or amongst SNPnet participants. Also, while the participants might follow and discuss a particular protocol that is said to target certain SNPs, other SNPs are also brought into the discussion, if not because of their possible relevance to the treatment protocol, then because of sub-forum participants' general interest in genetics.

That SNPs are relevant to the treatment of their symptoms has not been scientifically proven, however, and some participants on the sub-forum also doubt the validity of Yasko's protocol. One participant, for example, comments that many of Yasko's interpretations are 'completely unsupported by any research'. He is particularly concerned about claims made about 'random SNPs' that have no evidence of 'dysfunction associated with them'. In another thread, where the discussion turns towards Yasko's credentials, another participant adds: 'I guess that to get through this, I have to trust somebody along the way', while another comments: 'I cannot just trust one person's word'. What becomes clear from their discussions, however, is that while they at times question Yasko's work and the information they find online, they find support in each other's comments and stories, advice and suggestions, supported by links to various websites and participants' own data analyses.

DIY-style analysis tools are also used in the sense-making work. Participants have used a Google spreadsheet put together by a sub-forum participant to aid their translations. However, this has more recently been replaced by a software tool that analyses a person's 'raw' 23andMe data to produce what is called 'a methylation gene analysis'. Similar to the spreadsheet method—although now automated—the software will tell users which of the SNPs of interest to methylation are potentially problematic. The software colour-codes SNPs: red indicates a homozygous mutation (+/+); yellow indicates a heterozygous mutation ($\pm$); and green indicates that a user does not carry the specific mutation. It is suggested that users address the red and yellow SNPs. This is done by supplementation, e.g. of B12, B6 and folate. The software was developed by a sub-forum participant. However, on his own website, he emphasises that a website or report cannot determine what treatment or supplements a person needs. Instead, he suggests participants to individualise their treatments by 'listening to their bodies'. Others on the forum make similar suggestions. In the extract below, a forum participant responds to another participant's questions and comments about SNPs, and as the discussion moves on, she adds:

Get a basic feel for where you are when you add in simple stuff and take some time to learn this before you rush into anything. Hurrying usually ends up in crashing and lost time. [...] Remember, we do not know what you have been through or who you are, so this changes things too".

Jemma, SNPnet, posted 24 June 2013

The participant reminds others about the importance of their own illness biographies, where this kind of sharing of personal stories indeed becomes important because it provides context for the genetic data. It situates data in personal life stories, where it works as the basis for negotiation and advice, and it also reminds others that they are not alone. The sub-forum is not only a platform for collaborative sense-making where participants help to make sense of each other's data and give suggestions towards supplements and diets; through this sense-making work, they also provide support for each other. Participants respond to each other's stories and situations, and engage in dialogue, sharing links and analysis reports. Yet, because of the uncertainties, this biosensing practice comes to resemble an experiment that gets enacted in the space between the unknown and known of SNPs and life with a chronic illness. This is an experiment that involves not only materials and tools, but also the practice of 'listening to the body': an important concept put forward by SNPnet participants and repeated in conversations and discussions.

Making Sense of Ovulation

On Fertility Forums, women participate in discussions of what is happening to their bodies as well as to the bodies of others. Similar to participants on SNPnet, they ask questions, negotiate interpretations and share personal experiences, and through this interpretative work, they try to make sense of ovulation and fertility. While the ovulation biosensing devices are promoted as easy to use, for the users, the data they produce is not always easy to interpret. This interpretive work takes place through online exchanges in the form of 'collaborative coding', a term introduced by Julie Roberts (2012) in her analysis of four-dimensional (4D) ultrasound screening during pregnancy to describe the way in which sonographers, pregnant woman and their partners, friends or family narrate the imagery observed on the screen through coding themes such as family resemblances or foetal personality. Roberts argues that 4D images are not self-evident but instead depend on a coding process of social interaction and discourse in order to be meaningful. In ovulation biosensing, the concept of collaborative coding enables us to focus on the sense-making practices that women engage in, in order to understand the data they collect from biosensing devices. In particular, we focus on how collaborative coding enables women to decipher patterns observed in the microscope, to become more skilled in using the biosensing tools and to situate the body in and amongst different sets of data.

When making sense of ovulation biosensing data, women try to 'decipher' the patterns they observe in the device and to understand what these mean in relation to ovulation. In the case of the ovulation microscope, women describe how the patterns do not correspond to images or descriptions presented in the instruction sheet and thus seek support from women on the Fertility Forums, as in the case below:

MonsterMunching: I have been using a ferning microscope this cycle but have been finding it hard to analyse the pattern. I am getting close to Ov [Ovulation] and the pattern looks different than earlier in the month but it is not a ferning pattern. It is like a criss-cross pattern, like looking at a piece of material/weave under a microscope. Does anyone know if everyone gets a ferning pattern at O [ovulation]? Or can they look different? Can you O [ovulate] without a ferning pattern?

Stripeycracker: Hey, I found mine really confusing at first, but what I have since realised is that the slightest turn of the microscope part makes it look totally different - in my first month I didnt see any ferning, but then in my second I thought I just had the same again, until i turned the microscope the tiniest amount, and there were all the lines…I also found it hard at first to get the right amount on there - as too much or too little was not giving a sensible result - so sometimes I let it dry, and then tried again if the pattern wasn't clear.

Fertility Forum, accessed 15 January 2012

The user does not observe ferning patterns in the microscopic images but instead 'criss-crossing' or 'weaving'. Elsewhere in the forum, users describe *lint* or *spikeness,* lines may be *branchy* or *wavy,* dots may be described as *unconnected* or *partial,* they may be *bubbles, feathered particles* or *specs,* patterns may also be *good* or *lovely* and women also record *empty spaces.* The images that are presented in the microscope extend beyond that which is offered in the standardised instruction sheet, and women engage in the task of labelling in order to place their bodies within some framework of meaning.

In this sense, ovulation biosensing devices are more than 'peering technologies' (Hartouni 1997); they do not reveal that which cannot be seen through other means but, instead, construct ways of seeing. This can be observed more clearly in a post focusing on how the device is used. She advises fellow forum participants to focus on technique—on turning the microscope a tiny amount, of placing the right amount of saliva on the lens, of letting the saliva dry and repeating the action if sensible results are not achieved. The respondent shares her own experiences, but also guides other participants on how to 'do science' at home, carefully describing how each stage may facilitate or obstruct the visual field.

In the following example, a forum participant also requests advice on interpreting the image in the microscope, in relation to whether this is 'partial' or 'full ferning'.

StripeyZ: I've tried using the saliva scopes once before and couldn't get the hang of it. Now that I can get pictures of it, could you all have a look? Is this partial or full? They are different pictures of the same slide:

ChestnutsT: Full ferning. DTD! [do the deed/sexual intercourse]

StripeyZ: hooray! It was like that yesterday too! Also, my OPKs [Ovulation Predictor Kits/ovulation strips] aren't positive but they are distinctly darker than before. Should I take that as then being positive?

ChestnutsT: You're probably getting ready to ovulate… likely in the next day or two and likely get a positive opk in the next day. Do it… do it… do it… :)

StripeyZ: Still no positive OPK, and switched to partial ferning today. >:(

Sbean85: What cycle day are you on? Maybe your body geared up to ovulate but didn't? I would keep watching for ovulation and dtd as if you have confirmed ovulation. Hormones seem to come and go so quickly sometimes that it is hard to pin point exactly what's going on until the cycle is over.

Fertility Forum, accessed 10 November 2013

In this discussion, the participant receives different responses. One respondent confirms the patterns to be full ferning and advises sexual intercourse, although later suggests that the body is gearing up to ovulate, with this taking place within the next few days. Another respondent speculates that the body is prepared to ovulate but in fact did not. This participant recommends engaging in sexual activity regardless of the ferning patterns, emphasising the irregularity and unreliability of hormones. Although the women collaboratively code the ferning patters in relation to ovulation, there are few certainties provided by their responses. What emerges instead is a 'composite patchwork body' (Mol 2002) in which ferning is taking place but ovulation may not be, where hormones can be seen through the microscope but are also elusive—'coming and going'; where some tools do show changes but others do not; and where changes are a good sign but are simultaneously inconclusive.

This collaborative coding of ovulation biosensing data on online forums does not produce a decoded or fully known ovulating body but instead provides a space for women to engage in the uncertainties of the body in relation to ovulation and fertility, to try out, to experiment, to speculate and to deduce, and in some cases, to draw conclusions. These knowledge practices reveal a different way of coming to know the body, one that is sometimes messy, uncertain and laborious, yet highly traceable.

Knowing the Body: How and Where?

As health biosensors are increasingly moving outside the clinic and into commercial and online environments, they lead people into knowing their bodies in different ways, to the extent that the spatiality of body knowledge is changing. This does not mean that knowledge of the body is simply found in devices; rather, as users gather on online forums and engage in sense-making by doing, these biosensor networks become sites for doing knowledge in different ways with a focus on experimentation and exploration. Although measuring very different bodily events, both types of health biosensors involve this kind of experimentation, an experimentation that is always situated in personal biographies. This is sense-making by doing, in which forum participants review and discuss scientific and medical literature, convert data into other formats, observe and study patterns through mini-microscopes, and share 'practical knowledge' akin to how clinicians develop 'clinical knowledge' (Pols 2014).

Through this kind of experimentation characterised by uncertainty but also excitement and hope, users learn to have a biosensing body, and through this process of 'becoming affected', they get to know their bodies differently, to some extent. On SNPnet, this happens, for example, through becoming familiar with new words and concepts such as 'SNP' and 'methylation', and through the sharing of experiences that are turned into key concepts such as 'listening to the body' and 'go slow'. In the case of Fertility Forums, a different conception of ovulation and the body can be observed: one that is more open, irregular and uncertain. Yet, through the support and sense-making practices of the forums, the women manage and negotiate these uncertainties. In this context, those participants who know more about or who have more experience of a particular topic, or those who are able to contribute to a particular discussion also come to be seen as 'experts'. However, the authority and legitimacy which typically underpin modern medical institutions are not present here. Instead, new kinds of legitimacy and authority based on partiality, collaboration, uncertainty and *doings* begin to emerge.

Engaging in this kind of sense-making by doing, however, does not mean that medicine or clinical care has failed. Rather, the two biosensors as well as other personal medical devices (PMDs) present a kind of sense-making and support that often happens alongside clinical care.

As we have shown, support and care are indeed important processes involved in the kind of sense-making that happens on the forums. It is care, not as a product, but as a practice that meshes discussion, arte-facts, anticipations, body sensations and corporeal imaginaries. As participants engage in material practice, and as they share and discuss ovulation patterns and genetic susceptibilities, they also imagine their bodies in certain ways. It is through these networks of multiple and heterogeneous actors and processes that the biosensing body is consti-tuted and held together, and it is through the sense-making work that the participants learn to be affected in the Latourian sense. Therefore, while the health biosensors are promoted as direct-to-consumer prod-ucts and tools for 'self-knowledge', access to the meaning of the data generated thereby is anything but direct. The data might be consid-ered useful and actionable by the manufacturers, but as our two case studies have shown, it takes much work to make this data meaningful. Studying online forums is therefore in many ways an excellent way to critically analyse personal medical devices and how people make sense of and engage with the data that they generate outside of the clinical space. It offers a way to study what people actually do with the health biosensors and their data. How people will engage with health biosen-sors to understand their bodies cannot be known in advance; rather, it is in practice and by doing that people make sense of their biosensing data. Rather than consumers of health biosensors, individuals become participants in networks of biosensing, and it is through such networks that biosensing data becomes meaningful.

Yet, we cannot take for granted that the data will make sense—even after hard work. It might become what Nafus (2014) describes as 'dead data' or 'stuck data'. Therefore, as Nafus (2014, p. 208) argues, '[f]ar from producing certainty, sensor data often provokes a sense of vague-ness that is worked on until it becomes either clarity or action, failure or indifference'. Biosensing networks may, to some extent at least, protect users from this kind of failure, providing a form of caring relationality that 'helps' to reframe a relation to one's body, whether or not the data makes sense.

Notes

1. The notion of 'user' often comes with certain assumptions about who or what users are, but users come in many versions, and are not separate from the shaping of technologies (Oudshoorn and Pinch 2002).
2. Lancaster University Ethics Committee Approval was gained for the two studies on 23 May 2012 (Kragh-Furbo) and 20 July 2012 (Wilkinson).
3. By alternative medical practitioner, we mean practitioners who are not medical doctors, but who have certificates in alternative medicine and/or holistic health. For example, on Yasko's website, it says that '[t]his information is not intended to be substituted for consultation with a health care provider' (www.dramyyasko.com Yasko 2016).
4. It is important to note that this study has not focused on whether finding support online has been a response to a lack of clinical care or not.
5. See also Pols and Hoogsteyns (2016) on sharing of personal experiences on a web forum for people living with incontinence.

References

23andMe. (2015). What your DNA says about you. Available online at https://www.23andme.com/en-gb/. Accessed December 11, 2015.

Clarke, A., Shim, J., Mamo, L., Fosket, J., & Fishman, J. (2003). Biomedicalization: Technoscientific transformations of health, illness and U.S. biomedicine. *American Sociological Review, 68*(2), 161–194.

Crawford, K., Lingel, J., & Karppi, T. (2015). Our metrics, Our selves: A hundred years of self-tracking from the weight scale to the wrist wearable device. *Journal of European Cultural Studies, 18*(4–5), 479–496.

Duden, B. (1993). *Disembodying women: Perspectives on pregnancy and the unborn.* Cambridge, MA: Harvard University Press.

Epstein, S. (1995). The construction of lay expertise: AIDS activism and the forging of credibility in the reform of clinical trials. *Science, Technology and Human Values, 20*(4), 408–437.

Fiore-Gartland, B., & Neff, G. (2016). Disruption and the political economy of biosensor data. In D. Nafus (Ed.), *Quantified: Biosensing technologies in everyday life* (pp. 101–122). Cambridge, Mass: MIT Press.

Fox, N. (2015). Personal health technologies, micropolitics and resistance: A new materialist analysis. *Health.* doi:10.1177/1363459315590248.

Haraway, D. (1997). *Modest Witness@Second Millenium: Femaleman meets oncomouse feminism and technoscience* . London: Routledge.

Harris, A., Wyatt, S., & Kelly, S. (2013). The gift of spit (and the obligation to return it). *Information, Communication and Society, 16*(2), 236–257.

Hartouni, V. (1997). *Cultural conceptions: On reproductive technologies and the making of life.* Minneapolis: University of Minnesota Press.

Hine, C. (2008). Virtual ethnography: Modes, varieties, affordances. In N. Fielding, R. Lee, & G. Blank (Eds.), *The Sage handbook of online research methods* (pp. 257–270). London: Sage Publications.

Latour, B. (2004). How to talk about the body: The normative dimension of science studies. *Body and Society, 10*(2–3), 205–229.

Latour, B. (2005). *Reassembling the social: An introduction to actor-network-theory.* Oxford: Oxford University Press.

Law, J. (2009). Actor network theory and material semiotics. In S. Turner (Ed.), *The new blackwell companion to social theory* (pp. 141–158). Oxford: Blackwell Publishing Ltd.

Lupton, D. (2014). Beyond techno-Utopian: Critical approaches to digital health technologies. *Societies, 4,* 706–711.

Martin, A., Myers, N., & Viseu, A. (2015). The politics of care in technoscience. *Social Studies of Science, 45*(5), 625–641.

Markam, N. (2003). Representation in Online Ethnographies. A Matter of Context Sensitivity. Unpublished PhD Thesis. Department of Communication, University of Illinois at Chicago.

Mol, A. (2002). *The body multiple: Ontology in medical practice.* Durham, NC: Duke University Press.

Mort, M., Roberts, C., Furbo, M., Wilkinson, J., & Mackenzie, A. (2016). Biosensing: How citizens' views illuminate emerging health and social risks. *Health, Risk and Society* doi:10/1080/13698575.1135234.

Nafus, D. (2014). Stuck data, dead data and disloyal data: The stops and starts in making numbers into social practices. *Distinktion: Scandinavian Journal of Social Theory, 15*(2), 208–222.

Nafus, D. (Ed.). (2016). *Quantified: Biosensing technologies in everyday life.* Cambridge, Mass: MIT Press.

Novas, C., & Rose, N. (2000). Genetic risk and the birth of the somatic individual. *Economy and Society, 29*(4), 485–513.

Oudshoorn, N., & Pinch, T. (2002). *How users matter: The co-construction of users and technology.* Cambridge, Mass: MIT Press.

Pasveer, B. (1989). Knowledge of shadows: The introduction of X-ray images in medicine. *Sociology of Health & Illness, 11*(4), 360–381.

Pols, J. (2014). Knowing patients: Turning patient knowledge into science. *Science, Technology and Human Values, 39*(1), 73–97.

Pols, J., & Hoogsteyns, M. (2016). Shaping the subject of incontinence. Relating experience to knowledge. *ALTER, European Journal of Disability Research* 10 (2016), 40–53.

Puig de la Bellacasa, M. (2011). Matter of care in technoscience: Assembling neglected things. *Social Studies of Science, 41*(1), 85–106.

Rabeharisoa, V., Moreira, T., & Akrich, M. (2014). Evidence-based activism: Patients', users' and activists' groups in knowledge society. *BioSocieties, 9*(2), 111–128.

Roberts, J. (2012). 'Wakey, wakey baby': Narrating four dimensional (4D) bonding scans. *Sociology of Health & Illness, 34*(2), 299–314.

Rogers, R. (2013). *Digital methods.* Cambridge, Mass.: MIT Press.

Rose, N. (2007). *The politics of life itself. Biomedicine, Power, and Subjectivity in the twenty-first century.* New Jersey: Princeton University Press.

Till, C. (2014). Exercise as labour: Quantified self and the transformation of exercise into labour. *Societies, 4,* 446–462.

Viseu, A., & Suchman, L. (2010). Wearable augmentation: Imaginaries of the informed body. In J. Edwards, P. Harvey, & P. Wade (Eds.), *Technologized images, technologized bodies* (pp. 161–184). New York: Berghahn Books.

Yasko, A. (2004). *Autism: Pathways to recovery.* Bethel, ME: Neurological Research Institute.

Yasko, A. (2016). *Dr. Amy Yasko.* Available online at http://www.dramyyasko. com/. Accessed January 29, 2016.

4

In/Visible Personal Medical Devices: The Insulin Pump as a Visual and Material Mediator Between *Selves* and *Others*

Ava Hess

An image of the newly crowned Miss Idaho that surfaced on the internet in July 2014 had all the characteristics you might expect from a photograph of a beauty pageant swimsuit competition: flashy smile, thin figure, sparkly bikini, big hair and make-up. Upon closer inspection, something the approximate size and shape of an iPhone can be seen on her hip, attached to her skin with clear plastic tubing. The image went viral after being posted on Facebook by Miss Idaho herself, Sierra Sandison. 'There it is', opens her accompanying post and, with this simple statement, the insulin pump debuted on the big stage.

A. Hess (✉)
Independent Scholar, New York, NY, USA
e-mail: avakhess@gmail.com

© The Author(s) 2018
R. Lynch and C. Farrington (eds.), *Quantified Lives and Vital Data,*
Health, Technology and Society, https://doi.org/10.1057/978-1-349-95235-9_4

The 'Pumper' as Cyborg

An insulin pump is a small medical device about the size of a mobile phone that is worn on the body for twenty-four hours a day, every day. Whether hidden under clothing or worn visibly, this piece of technology accompanies its user to school, to bed, to work, on vacation and even possibly during sex or in the shower. The small machine communicates with the individual who wears it, sometimes loudly and sometimes through vibrations that can only be felt. It can be decorated with stickers, jewels or 'skins', and it may have been given a name or gender by the user. As far as medical devices are concerned, the insulin pump is especially personal. At the level of user interface, the continued entanglement of pump and person through a physical attachment between body and device complicates our tendency to differentiate between human and machine in traditional, dualistic terms. Donna Haraway suggests that 'for us, in imagination and other practice, machines can be prosthetic devices, intimate components, friendly selves' (1991, p. 178). Using the insulin pump as a case study, my focus is less on the 'imagination' than teasing out the extent to which 'other practice' can help to strengthen the affinity we share with our devices—an affinity that may also construct difference. Haraway's theoretical framework serves as a point of departure for this chapter, which ultimately argues that real-life cyborgs may complicate and blur boundaries between the human *self* and technological *other*, but equally that they also maintain or create such distinctions through everyday practices of use.

The cyborg has long been used to understand, and imagine, the relationship between humans and technology. This hybrid being of machine and organism has been championed by academia and popular culture alike as a deconstructive metaphor against dualistic understandings of the body/technology, natural/artificial or self/other. Such dualisms, argues Haraway, 'have all been systemic to the logics and practices of domination of women, people of color, nature, workers, animals—in short, domination of all constituted as others, whose task is to mirror the self' (1991, p. 177). Her essay 'A Cyborg Manifesto' (1991) outlines how a global paradigm shift in which the line between natural and artificial is blurred could lead to the dismantling of systemic oppression on a large scale. 'My cyborg myth', writes Haraway in defining her socialist feminist project, 'is about transgressed boundaries, potent fusions, and dangerous possibilities which progressive people might explore as one part of needed political work' (Haraway 1991, p. 154).

By linking so-called dualisms of self/other or culture/nature with systemic oppression, Haraway suggests that her cyborg myth not only has far-reaching implications but can also be enacted through our very own bodies and our relationships with non-human entities. Her corporeal language implies that change must occur on a personal level as well as a collective one: 'Why should our bodies end at the skin, or include at best other beings encapsulated by skin?' (1991, p. 178). While itself constructed as a 'myth', Haraway's work has still been criticised as 'curiously devoid of the singular material bodies' that she claims the cyborg metaphor represents (Seltin 2009, p. 51). Consideration of Haraway's cyborg myth in the PMD context demonstrates the value of examining the lived experience of those who are quite literally attached at the skin in terms of more fully fleshing out existing popular theories of hybridity in the social sciences.

Some decades ago, Arturo Escobar and colleagues advocated for ethnographic research that would help shed light on the degree to which technophilic, or technophobic, imaginings are 'in the process of becoming real' (1994, p. 214). Cyborg scholarship since then has seen a shift away from romanticised cyborg imagery and instead to 'our grandmother with a pacemaker' or other taken-for-granted biologically augmented people, drawing attention to the proliferation of everyday, real cyborgs among us (Gray 1995, p. 2). However, it is not only new technologies that make us cyborgs, as suggested by Marilyn Strathern (1988) who argues that people have always constituted hybrids by virtue of their social engagements with other human and non-human entities. Bruno Latour argues that in fact dualistic distinctions between nature and society are more constructed than literal; to Latour's *We Have Never Been Modern* (1993), insulin pump researcher Griet Scheldeman adds, 'we have always been cyborgs' (2010, p. 138).

And while PMDs become ever more ubiquitous in our daily lives, scholarship grows increasingly interested in how they may be contributing to the kinds of systemic oppression discussed by Haraway.

Investigations into how PMDs are designed, manufactured, regulated and circulated (e.g. see Kent and Bush, this volume; Faulkner, this volume) as well as the data they produce and how these are used (Dudhwala, this volume; Farrington, this volume; Till, this volume) suggest potential political or moral implications that may be otherwise taken for granted or obscured in our everyday use of them (Lynch, this volume; Smajdor and Stockl, this volume). While some of the contributions to this collection take a broader macro-level approach to PMDs in uncovering the wider networks that connect medicine and industry or domestic and/or international governance, the aim of this chapter is to narrow the focus onto the relationship between person and technology. I consider pump and pumper, and the day-to-day intimacies in which they are entangled, in order to demonstrate the value of drawing on material anthropological methodologies to understanding PMDs and the 'technological bodies' of those who rely on them. In Annemarie Mol's ethnography of the medical practices surrounding atherosclerosis in a Dutch hospital, she suggests that 'ontologies are brought into being, sustained, or allowed to wither away in common, day-to-day, sociomaterial practices' (Mol 2002, p. 6). Like Mol, I also focus on socio-material practices, foregrounding the body as well as the materiality of the insulin pump in a consideration of how its users navigate and construct the boundaries between *self* and *other* through their everyday practices.

The fluidity of bodily boundaries and the subject–object divide has been central to the ontological turn that has unfolded in the social sciences over the past few decades and especially in the field of Science and Technology Studies (STS), of which Mol and Haraway are both prominent scholars. But the so-called slogan of STS—it could be otherwise (Woolgar and Lezaun 2013, and see Matthewman this volume; Dudhwala, this volume)—reminds us of the impossibility of presuming bodies to be categorically open or permeable. These approaches suggest that people not only think differently about boundaries within and between bodies but that they also, through everyday practices, enact ontologies in which these distinctions are brought into being, with different practices enacting different bodies with different bodily boundaries. Such work also reinforces the notion that the self—itself not a static, immobile entity—is also not commensurate with a fixed, definitely bounded body.

Drawing primarily on ethnographic accounts of three women living with type 1 diabetes, I use the concept of in/visibilities to reflect the pump as an enigmatic object that can be seen on or felt through the body, while simultaneously being unseen and unfelt—sometimes separate to the body, at others literally incorporated. These case studies exemplify how individuals reconcile the tensions and contradictory impacts introduced by this PMD, which offers flexibility in travel, exercise and diet while limiting flexibility in other ways through its constant attachment to the body. A crucial question articulated in the beginning of the chapter is whether the dissolution of bodily boundaries between human and machine is necessary for personal well-being. I explore how the insulin pump[1] is felt on and through the individual body by examining strategies in how it is worn that help provide a necessary distinction between the 'diseased self' and the 'true self'. The relationship between person and pump inextricably informs the relationship between person with pump and other people, and it is this latter relationship that is of primary concern in the second half of the chapter. Personal identity is constantly shifting and negotiated through changing practices as a person with diabetes moves through different social and material environments. However, through such practices, boundaries between body and technology also shift, being at times dissolved and at times visible. The pump may be worn so that it is hidden, thereby de-emphasising a diabetic individual's differences, or it may be made more conspicuous through personalised decoration. I discuss how the pump, whose in/visibility can be manipulated, acts as a visual and material mediator in relationships between self and other. I conclude by returning briefly to Miss Idaho to suggest how the commonality and shared experience between people who have insulin pumps should not be taken for granted, but is actively and collaboratively constructed through these in/visibilities.

Researching Pumps and Pumping

For me, the insulin pump came into being as a far-off possibility and a vague clinical term, among many others, on the day I was diagnosed with type 1 diabetes. The nurses explained 'diabetes mellitus' as a term that actually refers to many different diseases, all of which involve a problematic relationship between the body and insulin, a hormone produced by cells in the pancreas. In some kinds of diabetes, like type 2, the body is unable to use insulin or to create enough of it. In 'your' diabetes, as I was told, the body attacks the cells that make insulin so that you effectively have none at all. I would have to depend on synthetic insulin to survive, using syringes and insulin pens to inject or 'give shots' multiple times a day, including whenever I ate foods containing carbohydrates. Eventually, they said, I might choose to go on a pump. Four years later, I did.

As someone who has diabetes and uses a pump myself, the autoethnographic[2] nature of my project fundamentally shaped the form that my research took. While clearly acknowledging that I was also conducting research in this field, over the course of a year I participated in online forums and social media sites dedicated to diabetes, took part in weekly Tweetchats and attended social meet-ups for pumpers in addition to conducting interviews by phone, email and in person. My participants shared freely in what often became more intimate conversations than the semi-structured interviews I had planned for. Of the three participants whose interviews have laid the foundations for this chapter, two responded to my call for participants that I circulated via email and social media to groups for people living with diabetes. The third was a young woman named Evie[3] whom I had met before I began conducting research, on the recommendation of our common nurse at the local diabetes centre in Oxfordshire. At the time, I was considering transferring to a particular pump that Evie had recently begun using and she kindly offered to share her experience with me. In many ways, the three participants whose experiences are discussed here amount to a very narrow proportion of the larger population of people who have type 1 or who use insulin pumps: all three are white, professional women living in the UK with above-average access to resources. On the other hand, the experiences and viewpoints of these three women represent key variations and examples of practices around insulin pumps, resonating with the wider range of sentiments I found expressed across online forums.

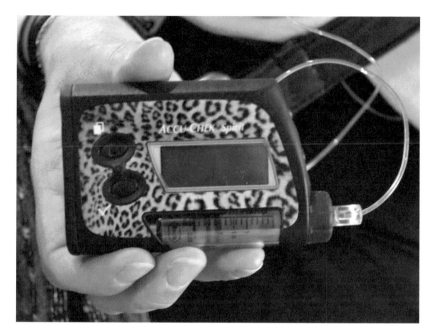

Fig. 4.1   Accu-chek pump with leopard print sticker

Each of these participants uses a different kind of pump, and between them, they cover three of the most commonly used models. Those made by Animas, Medtronic or Roche (Fig. 4.1) are of the conventional, tubed type: the main unit that houses the insulin is rectangular, approximately the size of a deck of cards, with about 20–40 inches of thin, flexible plastic tubing. A disposable infusion set connects the pump to the body, often on the abdomen, by using a needle to puncture the skin and insert the tiny plastic tube or cannula through which insulin is delivered 4–8 millimetres beneath the skin. After the insertion, the needle is removed but the cannula and adhesive mount stay in place for 2–3 days until the infusion site must be changed to avoid infection. So while the pump and its flexible plastic tubing can be removed if one is, for example, changing or showering, the infusion set will remain in place on the body. While the Animas pump is completely waterproof and has the clearest screen, the Roche model has a meter-remote that

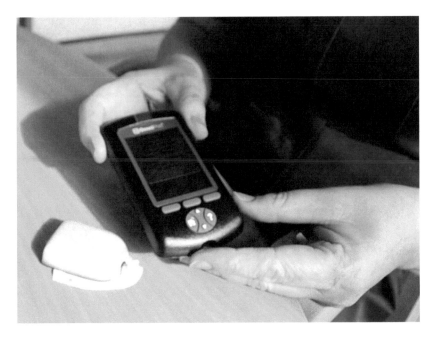

Fig. 4.2 The OmniPod system

can control the pump from a distance. Sierra Sandison, the beauty pageant winner, uses a pump made by Tandem that has a touchscreen display similar to popular smartphones. The OmniPod is rather different from these devices and is approximately a quarter of the size. It uses a similar needle mechanism to insert the cannula, but the pump itself comes on an adhesive mount that attaches directly to the body instead of using separate infusion sets and tubing. These tubeless, disposable 'pods' must be operated by a separate device called a Personal Diabetes Manager which also serves as a blood glucose testing device (Fig. 4.2).[4]

As of 2015, there are an estimated 415 million people (aged between 20 and 70 years old) living with diabetes worldwide. In high-income countries such as the UK, 7–12% of all people living with diabetes are estimated to have type 1 (International Diabetes Federation 2015, p. 34). Clear numbers of those using insulin pumps are hard to come by, since the corporations that make these devices are not required to share this information. However, estimates in 2014 suggested that there were around 0.75–1 million people using insulin pumps worldwide, with the percentage of people with type 1 diabetes that turn to insulin pump therapy increasing significantly with every year (Heinemann et al. 2015). When needles are used to administer insulin, a person must inject both a long-acting insulin that should last around 24h and fast-acting insulin used to counteract meals or to correct elevated blood glucose levels. The insulin pump more closely mimics a functioning pancreas through the use of only fast-acting insulin. The insulin is released in micro-doses through a continuous but adjustable 'basal' rate, with user-prompted 'boluses' given for meals and corrections. Insulin pump therapy is widely believed to provide better management and tighter control over type 1 diabetes than multiple daily injections; it has been officially recommended in the treatment of eligible patients by healthcare authorities such as the National Institute for Health and Care Excellence (NICE) in the UK, which stated in its recommendation that insulin pumps not only to provide better health but also an 'enhancement in quality of life' (NICE 2008). Clinical research findings (e.g. Grunberger et al. 2014) have also demonstrated that insulin pump therapy helps to lower hemoglobin A1c, a blood test commonly used to assess glycaemic control in patients with diabetes.[5] By allowing users to adjust insulin doses spontaneously and precisely, pumps provide more flexibility when travelling, exercising and eating—or not eating—as desired. In other ways, the flexibility offered by the pump is severely limited as a treatment in which the patient is, quite literally, tethered to another entity. However, it is not the flexibility of the pump as treatment that I focus on here, but rather the socio-material practices it allows. In this context, the insulin pump emerges as a marker and a mediator between body and non-body and between self and others, making itself and the presence of diabetes in/visible.

The Absent Pump

Ultimately, my participants saw bodily awareness of the pump as decreasing over time and often located this unawareness within certain sensory modalities or body parts. Evie, a research professional in her twenties, suggested she no longer felt the weight of the OmniPod on her arm in the same way she used to and would even forget its location on her body: 'sometimes when I'm taking off trousers I'll think, "don't hit the pump," but actually I'm not wearing it there, it's on my arm'. Or, in response to a question about the noises her pump makes, Patricia, another interviewee who uses a Roche Accu-Chek pump, referred to the sound of pumping insulin as the '"ch-ch-" noise you ignore most of the time'. All three women also agreed that anxieties felt about the insulin pump before transitioning to pump therapy dissipated to one degree or another upon starting, further indicating the body's ability to physically overcome human–machine dualisms. The third interviewee whose comments I draw on is Allison, a current user of an Animas pump for whom the 'novelty has well worn off' after 18 years of pumping. She volunteers at a charity that supports patients in accessing diabetes technologies, and gives the following advice to people hesitant about starting pump therapy because of negative reviews or scary stories they see online: 'it's like your teeth: if your teeth are working fine, you don't post on Facebook "today my teeth feel excellent, I've just eaten a lovely meal and I chewed every mouthful" but if you have a toothache you're like "ow, give me sympathy!" You write it on Facebook. So the fact that the pump works most of the time and makes daily life possible is something we get to take for granted'.

In her own words, Allison more or less explains physician-philosopher Drew Leder's concepts of 'experiential disappearance' and 'incorporation'. Leder's use of the term 'the absent body' refers to the body's tendency to disappear from consciousness in daily life until prompted to 'dys-appear', or reemerge problematically in response to physical or social stimuli (1990, p. 84). Bodily 'incorporation' of tools or skills functions in a parallel way: 'Heidegger notes that the "ready-to-hand" tool withdraws insofar as it functions unproblematically. Only when the tool manifests a certain "un-readiness-to-hand" by virtue of becoming unusable, missing, or standing in the way, must we take explicit account of it' (Leder 1990, p. 32). When technological devices, like insulin pumps, become incorporated into the body, they 'disappear from view, they recede into the background, become tacit' by virtue of repetitive use (Scheldeman 2010, p. 154). Understanding the body as open in this way allows for the conceptualisation of how the pump, and the diabetes it signifies, can be 'forgotten'.[6]

But the opposite is also the case. Patricia, a single woman in her fifties, works as an analyst in a retail chain and has been pumping for just over a year. The day before we met, she had been given a cortisone injection for a tendon injury in her wrist. Because cortisone is known to increase insulin resistance and therefore elevate blood sugar, Patricia raised her basal rate, which also meant she had to check her blood sugar more frequently to avoid dropping too low. When having insulin injections, without the ability to adjust the amount of long-acting insulin once the daily injection has been given, she stated that 'you just let it be'. When using the pump, alternatively, she stated that 'you have more options to change things, so you do, and then that's more considerations … Now I'm more conscious more of the time that I'm Type 1'.[7]

How then might researchers reconcile the simultaneous in/visibility of the pump and of diabetes, and how are these contradictions reconciled in the daily lives of the people who live with them? (I am, of course, both researcher and reconciler.) In their study of hypoglycaemia, Annemarie Mol and John Law suggest that the ability to prevent or counteract low blood sugar depends on the incorporation of non-human entities through practices like measuring blood sugar or eating an apple (2004, p. 51). Whereas in this example personal medical well-being is at stake rather than the global political well-being of Haraway's cyborg myth, there are striking similarities in how both are achieved: 'machines can only be instruments if the body can manipulate and incorporate them. So measuring depends on an open rather than an isolated body. The actively measuring body merges with its measuring machines' (Mol and Law, *ibid.*). If we accept that different 'well-beings' exist for different people (see, e.g. Corsín-Jimenez 2007), then surely they are pursued through different creative engagements and practices. Mol and Law suggest that a body must merge with machines to manipulate and incorporate them, but this leaves us wondering what this merging looks and feels like, how it is achieved, and how much is required for different human–machine relationships. The examination of personal medical devices here—insulin pumps and their more permanent attachments to one's person—questions whether the body must *always* 'merge with' or 'incorporate' machines to achieve well-being. Instead, these data suggest that the creative pursuit of well-being takes an alternate path, one in which boundaries between the (human) *self* and (technological) *other* are not only blurred but also remade through everyday situated socio-material practices.

Pumphrey

Evie, like other participants, did not want to go on an insulin pump at first. Unlike some, she was not prompted to start because she felt that her diabetes had become out of control. Still, she took the opportunity offered by her diabetes nurse to take a conventional-style, tubed pump home for the weekend to wear and practice 'pumping' with saline. She recalled that, after that first weekend, 'I didn't really look back and it all just became instantly a part of me'. Evie is lighthearted and comfortable sharing embarrassing stories or the more intimate aspects of wearing a pump, for example, in her 'knickers' or while having sex, with our common experience as pumpers perhaps making these open exchanges possible. For Evie, her first pump had a gender (male) and for some time she referred to 'him' by his name, 'Pumphrey'. 'As time went on I did that less', she explained: 'it became so much more of me. It was less of Pumphrey and it was more of just an extra arm or something. I was so used to it being on me it wasn't as if I was wearing anything … it submerged with me physically'. After Pumphrey's warranty expired, Evie used it as an opportunity to test out a different kind of pump, the OmniPod. When I first met her, she had just switched a few weeks earlier and wondered whether she would build up a 'connection' with the Personal Diabetes Manager meter-remote or see it as a 'replacement pump' in any way. Several months later, Evie no longer thought this would be possible, but welcomed the change:

> I think [the Omnipod] is helpful for me because it helps me conceptualize the diabetes. [Diabetes is] very much a part of my life and part of who I am but if I can just dispose of the OmniPod it's like it's still external to me. I'd be kidding myself if I tried to say that diabetes is

separate…I think about it all the time, you have to. But because I can dispose of the OmniPod, it's like I can still brush it off, start again with something new. It's a bit cathartic. Get rid of it, put a new one on, it's clean, it's fresh, I'm not building up an attachment with it, it's not taking over my life whereas a pump might do that. Sometimes with the pump—the other one—it was like that came first. It was like, 'it doesn't want to sit there' or 'I'm wearing these clothes but it can't go there, I've got to change my outfit' but with the OmniPod it's more of a mutual relationship. It's there to help me but also I can just pull the brakes, take it off, change it.

Evie's pump history began with the pump as an entity defined in clear distinction from her by virtue of its separate name and gender. Leder's suggestion that 'in its use of tools and machines the body supplements itself through annexing artificial organs' (1990, p. 30) can be seen quite literally in how Evie's body incorporated Pumphrey 'like an extra arm'. Pumphrey's experiential invisibility and incorporation into the body were, however, seen negatively rather than positively, leading her to take proactive measures in changing to a treatment that involved different daily practices.

If 'objects come into being—and disappear—with the practices in which they are manipulated' (Mol 2002, p. 5), then Mol suggests that reality multiplies and more than one 'diabetes' can exist. Not only does wearing a technological device as opposed to injecting insulin make us live a different diabetes, but the diabetes that comes into being by wearing an OmniPod as opposed to another pump can be wholly different as well. As Lucy Norris writes in regard to another wearable object—clothing—'objects and persons are things in the process of becoming in relation to each other, and are perceived as participating in an ongoing continual transformation in the inter-artefactual domain' (2004, p. 69).

The OmniPod requires a routine that allowed Evie to maintain a desirable amount of distance from her diabetes. And, while she understands diabetes as an all-encompassing disease that is not 'separate' from her, she still objectifies it in the form of its treatment—the pods—over which she feels she has more control. Control is central to anthropologist Michael Jackson's understanding of the human–technology interface. He argues that 'our relationships with both persons and machines will depend upon the degree to which we feel in control of these relationships, as well as the degree to which these relationship [sic] are felt to augment rather than diminish our own sense of wellbeing' (2002, p. 336). For Evie, her well-being depended directly on the amount of control she felt she had in the relationship with her pump, which increased from one in which Pumphrey was 'taking over' to the 'mutual relationship' she had with the OmniPod.

Jackson further argues that the more an individual feels in control over a machine, the more it is incorporated and understood as part of the self (2002); Evie's account provides a different perspective, one in which the more *other* the pump became, the more control she was able to feel. Jackson develops his arguments in the context of the interrelationships between humans and machines intersubjectively, with analyses of Gameboys, CT scanners, computers and allotransplantation contributing to his theory. Evie's pump switch suggests, however, that an appreciation for the differentiation between technologies and their nuanced materialities can provide insight into incorporations of different kinds. As technology becomes obsolete at an increasingly rapid rate, the insulin pump will soon be replaced by integrated closed-loop systems and the artificial pancreas (see Farrington, this volume for accounts from research participants using this latter technology), perhaps creating further varying senses of control and of the self.

Out of Sight, Out of Mind

In one of our conversations, Evie described diabetes as 'the unseen disability'; except in cases of extreme low or high blood sugar, there are no symptoms that manifest externally.[8] 'Going on to a pump was very much a change in the fact that I would have to show people', Evie began to say before quickly interrupting herself: '…that was just in my head—when I got a pump I could actually hide it quite effectively'. When prompted to discuss the transition from injections to using a pump, interviewees recalled having anxieties about its conspicuous appearance. But in all cases this anxiety dissipated to some degree once they actually began pumping.

By changing from a conventional pump model to the tubeless pods, Evie took rather drastic measures to ensure what she felt was the right amount of separation between herself and her pump, but similar boundaries are drawn in more mundane, everyday actions as well. Patricia, for example, would sometimes remove an infusion set from her stomach and insert a new one on her lower back instead. Motioning to the front of her body, she explained that she likes not having anything 'there': 'You look down on and you're just you. Sounds a bit perverse but you know when you're in the shower and you've not got things stuck to you? Or you have but you can't see it, so maybe I'm just fooling myself—well I am because it's on my bum!'

Notably, although the senses do not work independently and cannot be easily distinguished from one another (see, e.g. Howes 2005), discomfort with the attachment of the pump is dominated by a different sensory modality in the experiences of Evie and Patricia: Evie's discomfort was described as primarily tactile and Patricia's as visual. In Leder's terms (1990), the pump dys-appears for Patricia when it is seen. Just like the 'absent body', the pump spends most of its time outside corporeal consciousness, and for Patricia, 'it's only when you go to the loo or something and see the tubing' that it reappears. The pump's incorporation into the body allows Patricia to forget its presence. As such, choosing a pump model that is fully controllable by meter-remote was crucial as it allows her to 'forget' while still maintaining her health and giving herself insulin. The meter-remote enables the pump's invisibility in the everyday since, as Patricia explained, 'I put my pump wherever I'm going to put it in the morning and I don't look at it again all day'. Only through sight is she made aware of the pump and then takes active measures to not see it. For example, she would sometimes 'feel it to make sure it's not sticking out' of her clothing before she has even noticed the pump or tubing visually. Such practices suggest that Patricia was able to maintain a view of herself as a body separate to her pump; the shared boundary between body and medical device technology became less troublesome if she could not see it.

Much of this discussion centres around active measures taken on behalf of the user to render the pump 'invisible', either to the self or others. This is by no means to suggest that the visibility or invisibility of the pump is a matter of personal choice. Diabetes may be an invisible disability, so to speak, but the purpose of most diabetes-related technologies is to make it more apparent, e.g. blood glucose changes within the body externalised through alarms that are activated by a continuous glucose monitor in order to prompt action by the user. Across websites, forums and interviews, both people who have the illness and their loved ones express a widespread frustration and disappointment that, given the advanced state of medical innovation, devices used to monitor or treat diabetes are not more miniature, user-friendly or aesthetic in design. This sentiment is also easily discernible in casual comments by healthcare professionals, including diabetes nurses, endocrinologists and even product representatives themselves. However, while many aspects of living with diabetes are out of patients' control (e.g. how sickness or hormonal changes can have unexpected effects on blood glucose), there is also room for agency and creativity with respect to the available technologies and the ways in which these may be drawn on to construct one's own body and embodiment of diabetes. The transition to pump therapy, to borrow from Scheldeman, 'is not just a matter of using a pump to treat diabetes, but of a different modality of embodiment and thus a different way of being-in-the-world' (2010, p. 157). Felt or corporeal in/visibilities are examples of how the pump allows for differing ways of being-in-the-world, whether these technologies are seen or unseen by others. The pump, rather than radically transcending or anchoring divisions within and between people, acts as a material and visual mediator within the relationships in which people with diabetes find themselves.

Pumps, Others and Otherness

Insulin pumps, by virtue of their particular materialities, are both restrictive and allow a flexibility in how they can be worn by the body, affecting not only how they are perceived by pumpers themselves but by others as well. While each participant had her own particular preferences for how to wear the pump, they all shared a common goal of striking a balance between practicality and discreteness. Diverse strategies had to be used to accommodate the specificity of each pump model and the types of clothing required by different places and occasions. Conventional pumps with tubing could be worn in pockets of jeans, although this was not possible in work trousers, which often do not have pockets. Suppliers often provide a clip with these pumps for external attachment to clothing but Allison, the only participant who used one, attached it to her waistline so that it was unnoticeable under her shirt; other participants complained that clips made the pump even more bulky and likely to be noticed. Some people wore elastic armbands, garters or Spibelts that held the pump, but these could only be accommodated by certain outfits. Moreover, visibility was not the sole concern. Though many women wear the pump in their bra, Evie explained her decision not to do this since someone might be able to feel it while hugging her—thus, what is felt as well as seen by others is also a concern. With the design of each new pump, a shifting set of tensions in the form of restrictions and flexibilities is introduced. The OmniPod, for example, can be worn on more places on the body (including the arms, thighs and even chest), but its position can only be changed every three days, unlike conventional pumps whose tubing allows for easy rearrangement according to outfit changes.

Within the context of the constraints presented by a chronic medical condition, the pump is inflexible in its physicality in as much as it externalises a function of the internal body. And yet the (relative) flexibility afforded by its material particularities allows the pumper a degree of control over the circumstances in which their diabetes becomes known by others. When Patricia and I first met in a busy café in central London, she comfortably took her pump out of the Spibelt from underneath her shirt to show me. But this is not how she is in every situation or with everyone: 'Regardless of the pump, I don't want to be *the* diabetic. I don't want that to define me when I first meet somebody. Definitely at work if I'm with suppliers, none of them would know that I was type 1 and I wouldn't want them to know'. By using her pump only before or after work meetings, Patricia was able to manipulate the apparent visibility of her treatment and her illness or *otherness*.

Expounding Lacan's understanding of the 'gaze', Simon Cohn explains the paradox of seeing as 'a process emanating from the actor to the object, yet [which] also can be conceptualised as an equivalent process of the object making itself apparent to the actor' (2007, p. 98). Patricia curbs the pump's ability to make itself visible to her (i.e. by moving infusion sets from her front) but also to others (i.e. keeping it from sticking out of clothing). In the shower, or other moments when the pump *dys-appears*, the pump as object actively participates in the dual process described by Cohn. In visual encounters with other people, it is the body-as-object that manipulates how it is seen, to some degree, by making the pump visible or invisible. That the body, as an object of the gaze, can actively intervene into how it is seen is made possible by the phenomenon of perception as being both through and of the body. As Merleau-Ponty writes, 'the enigma is that my body simultaneously sees and is seen. That which looks at all things can also look at itself and recognise, in what it sees, the "other side" of its power of looking. It sees itself seeing' (1964, p. 162). It is the body's ability to perceive the world as a subject that makes it aware of its simultaneous existence as an object. The effort put into arranging the pump differently reflects not only a self-awareness that one can be seen but also that the way one is seen has significant social implications.

'Arguably the true challenge is not simply a recognition of the impossibility of dividing the body from the self, or the self from the social', suggests Cohn in discussing patients with type 2 diabetes, 'but that humans are, through technologies of symbolism, reflexive. This, then, enables individuals to project a sense of themselves, of the world and, crucially, their own place in it' (2013, p. 194). For people with diabetes, the pump itself can constitute one of these 'technologies of symbolism;' it both enables reflection of what does or does not count as part of the self and, as a visual and material mediator in social relations, enables a projection of the self to others. The pump often comes to objectify diabetes, enabling the disease to be conceptualised as separate from the self as in Evie's case, or even forgotten altogether. The pump involves a new way of being-in-the-world that makes the individual bear difference physically, as Patricia states: 'when you're on injections, you're only different when you inject, whereas now I carry it around with me'. As Cohn notes for people who are chronically ill, and I would add, people with wearable medical devices, 'it becomes increasingly difficult to maintain a distinction between the diseased and the true self' (2013, p. 209). If, at some times, the body perceives the pump as other than the self, therein lies the possibility that other people will see the pump in this way too. The pump is at once *other* than the self and a marker of the self's *otherness*.

Rane Willerslev suggests that in visual encounters with an other, the 'enigma' of perception described by Merleau-Ponty becomes particularly crucial: 'this self-reflexive or mirror-sense of vision is … strikingly necessary as a kind of defence mechanism against the dissolution of the self in relations where people steer a difficult course between transcending difference and maintaining identity' (2007, p. 41). Pumpers steer this difficult course daily in not wanting to be '*the* diabetic' but at the same time unable, from a medical perspective, to be in denial of their diabetes altogether. If, as Willerslev suggests, the self-reflexivity implied in vision allows for the navigation or balance of these two, we might begin to understand what role the pump plays. By nature of its in/visibility, which Patricia was able to manipulate to some degree, the pump acts as a mediator between Patricia's so-called true self and her diabetes. Through making her pump invisible to herself in various ways, she enabled its experiential disappearance, using the meter-remote to sustain her health while also maintaining a sense of self as separate from the diabetes it lives with.

The pump's in/visibility also mediates pumpers' social relationships. By keeping her pump invisible to the people she worked with, Patricia was able to de-emphasise any difference between herself and her co-workers by keeping her pump invisible to them, thereby allowing her to assert parts of her self-identity other than her diabetes. Positioning one's self-identity as close to those of peers can also be achieved through non-visual manipulations of the pump, as Patricia explained: 'I have all sounds and alarms turned off on mine. I don't want to be the beeping person in the corner of the office'. Ironically, the best strategy for downplaying differences can also be acknowledging them directly and moving on, as when Patricia has to use her pump at a restaurant and explains what she is doing rather than risk social alienation or offending others in being mistaken for texting at the table. Evie described using a similar strategy which could potentially backfire: 'occasionally I'd draw attention to it and say, "that's my OmniPod. It's just ticking, don't worry about it", and people say "we've not even heard it"'. In this example, the limits of the 'enigma' of perception are made clear, making explicit the corporeal distances between people.

Whereas in these contexts the pump was de-emphasised through practice to achieve commonality, at other times it is manipulated to emphasise visible differences. When I asked Patricia how she would characterise her relationship with her pump, her first response was that the Accu-Chek pump she has 'is the ugliest pump. It just comes in black'. She followed this by showing me her solution: leopard-print stickers (Fig. 4.1). In describing her sticker collection, Patricia repeatedly stressed two ways in which decorating changed her relationship with her pump. 'As soon as I stuck it on, it became *mine*', she said, hinting at the process by which an 'ugly' and impersonal commodity-like object can be made inalienable through active, creative consumption (see, e.g. Miller 2001). The second consequence of this visual personalisation was primarily social, providing a subject for conversation and a point of comparison between her and other pumpers. She described social meet-ups with other pumpers where their device accessories might be shown off, prompting questions about what they are, how they work or where to get them. Here, Patricia's concern is not so much about being '*the* diabetic', but of not being just one of many people living with diabetes. 'If I put it on a table with everyone else's, it's still *mine*', she said, suggesting that in drawing visual attention to her pump, Patricia balances an achievement of commonality with an assertion of her own unique self.

Pump stickers as a topic occupied a great deal of my interview with Patricia, coming as a surprise to us both. Patricia prefaced statements about customising her pump with disparaging remarks: 'I know it sounds really stupid but …' However, it clearly seemed important to her and, in fact, to the pumping community at large. Tips and examples of pump accessories or decorations are commonly shared on personal or group social media accounts, online forums and Tweetchats.

Considering visual-material transformations of the pump—and the proliferation of posts about them—within the context of Alfred Gell's anthropological theories of art suggests they are far from trivial.

For Gell, art is 'a system of action, intended to change the world rather than encode symbolic propositions about it' (1998, p. 6). As such, the study of art requires an action-centred approach that is 'preoccupied with the practical mediatory role of art objects in the social process rather than with the interpretation of objects "as if" they were texts'—or in other words, an approach that asks what art does rather than what it means (*ibid*). Far from being merely passive or symbolic objects, stickers add to the pump's own capacity for mediation, actively involving Patricia in more social relations. Customised pumps do more than signify a desire to maintain a sense of self; as the 'congealed residue of performance and agency in object-form', they actively contribute to the construction of identity, not just its representation (Gell 1998, p. 68). Leopard-print stickers, bejewelled OmniPods or pump 'skins' bring the pumper into a world where some amount of control is maintained, despite the 'uncontrollable' elements that diabetes inevitably brings to her life.

Making a Cyborg Body

For decades, Haraway has urged feminists to consider building coalitions based on affinity rather than a so-called shared or given identity. And though a beauty queen seems a highly unlikely candidate to embody Haraway's cyborg myth in the flesh, echoes of Haraway's project (1991) can be seen in Sierra Sandison's Facebook post. After publicly sharing the photograph of herself as Miss Idaho on Facebook, Sierra Sandison initiated the hashtag #showmeyourpump to encourage fellow pumpers to post photographs of themselves with their devices to social media. This message to her online audience is intended to amass solidarity and result in collective action; she writes that challenges like diabetes or insulin pumps can be used to 'not only empower yourself and grow as an individual, but to serve and influence other people as well'. The response to Sandison's request was overwhelming, and more and more 'pump selfies' are still shared every day.

Pump selfies join other diabetes-related material on the web that presumes the existence of a commonly shared 'diabetic experience'. While these popular memes, inside jokes and anecdotal posts may claim to articulate a singular experience of diabetes, my data suggests the experience of diabetes not only differs between individuals but can be constructed differently by the same person in different contexts and through different socio-material practices. Mol and Law propose that, at the level of the individual, 'the assumption that we *have* a coherent body or *are* a whole hides a lot of work' (2004, p. 57). Through this chapter, some of the work that my interviewees undertook has been brought out, with participants continually 'making' their diabetic bodies in different ways and, following Mol, making different diabetes. While such differences do not reflect a common experience of diabetes, pump selfies allow a means of constructing a shared diabetes through person, pump and photograph. The pump selfie movement—with its crowned, and tethered, mascot—simultaneously resists normative beauty standards of the pure and able-bodied while creating its own normalising discourse on diabetes pumps that *should* be seen. This narrative implies that making the pump (and therefore diabetes) visible is empowering and helps to build a collective, whereas a focus on the everyday practices of people with diabetes suggests rather that the ability to choose when, where, how and in front of whom the pump is made visible is more important to individuals.

Material and sensory anthropology, by considering the complex interrelationships between people and objects (e.g. Jackson 2002; Strathern 1988), has enabled a 'critique of the self-enclosed, clearly bounded individual [that] examines how the borders and boundaries between subjects are porous and permeable, meaning that the limits of the body are not defined by the skin for example' (Blackman 2008, p. 65). Boundaries of the body are created and maintained, as well as blurred and complicated, through the practices and actions in which persons and objects are mutually implicated. This is not to suggest a return to taking the 'troubling dualisms' described by Haraway for granted as natural or given, but to ensure against the 'tendency to presume, rather than ask, what a body is and where its significant boundaries are located' (Taylor 2005, p. 749). While focusing here at the level of the individual, there is space for further work on how the collective and networked 'body' of the insulin pumper is made, both online and offline, by the diabetes community at large.

Notes

1. This approach brings together different sorts of pumps which function in similar ways. These are grouped together as if these were one object within biomedical discourses, but of course the term 'wearable insulin pumps' refers to a range of different devices with different materialities and affordances.
2. I refer here to Hayano's (1979) understanding of the term as an insider's account of a group to which the self as researcher belongs.
3. All participants are referred to by pseudonym.
4. A common misconception is that insulin pumps monitor blood glucose and adjust insulin doses automatically. Though closed-loop artificial pancreas systems are currently undergoing clinical trials (see Farrington, this volume) and companies are increasingly integrating their pumps with continuous blood glucose monitors, at the time of publication all pumps on the market except the Medtronic MiniMed 670G must still be prompted by the user to give insulin for blood sugar corrections or carbohydrate intake.
5. Because insulin pumps are used primarily in the treatment of type 1 diabetes, I hereafter use the term 'diabetes' to refer specifically to this type unless otherwise noted.
6. See Scheldeman's (2010) study of young pumpers in Scotland for a different concern arising with regard to pumps, i.e. how the pump allowed her teenaged participants to 'forget' their diabetes, thereby leading to more infrequent use of the pump and consequently deteriorating health.
7. Patricia's statement resonates with one of the earliest studies of adults on a 'first-generation' pump. In 1981, after 15 patients at Guy's Hospital Medical School in London completed a three-week pump therapy trial, Dr. Pickup and his fellow colleagues reported that, 'Many patients remarked that the treatment made them more aware of being a diabetic, which they usually regarded unfavourably' (Pickup et al. 1981, p. 767).

8. Using Goffman's (2009) definitions of stigma, Balfe and Jackson argue that university students living with diabetes have a 'discreditable stigma', one that does not 'continually display a visible sign of their dissimilarity from "normals" if kept under control' (2007, p. 782). The diabetes technologies used are simultaneously in/visible in that they both enable stigma to be 'discreditable' by keeping diabetes under control and also threaten to make it obvious or 'discredited' if noticed.

Acknowledgements All interview material used in this chapter was gained with informed consent and is used with permission.

References

Balfe, M., & Jackson, P. (2007). Technologies, diabetes and the student body. *Health and Place., 13*(4), 775–787.

Blackman, L. (2008). *The body: The key concepts*. London: Berg.

Cohn, S. (2007). Seeing and drawing: the role of play in medical imaging. In C. Grasseni (Ed.), *Skilled visions: between apprenticeship and standards* (pp. 91–105). Oxford: Berghahn.

Cohn, S. (2013). Being told what to eat: Conversations in a diabetes day centre. In P. Caplan (Ed.), *Food, health and identity* (pp. 193–212). London: Routledge.

Corsin-Jimenez, A. (Ed.). (2007). *Culture and well-being. Anthropological approaches to freedom and political ethics*. London: Pluto Press.

Escobar, A., Hess, D., Licha, I., Sibley, W., Strathern, M., & Sutz, J. (1994). Welcome to Cyberia: Notes on the anthropology of cyberculture [and comments and reply]. *Current Anthropology, 35*(3), 211–231.

Gell, A. (1998). *Art and agency: An anthropological theory*. Oxford: Clarendon Press.

Goffman, E. (2009). *Stigm: Notes on the management of spoiled identity*. New York: Touchstone.

Grunberger, G., Abelseth, J., Bailey, T., Bode, B., Handelsman, Y., Hellman, R., et al. (2014). Consensus statement by the American Association of Clinical Endocrinologists/American College of Endocrinology insulin pump management task force. *Endocrine Practice*.

Gray, C. (1995). *The cyborg handbook*. London: Routledge.

Haraway, D. (1991). *Simians, cyborgs, and women: The reinvention of nature.* New York: Free Association Books.

Hayano, D. (1979). Auto-ethnography: paradigms, problems, and prospects. *Human Organization, 38*(1), 99–104.

Heinemann, L., Fleming, G., Petrie, J., Holl, R., Bergenstal, R., & Peters, A. (2015). Insulin pump risks and benefits: a clinical appraisal of pump safety standards, adverse event reporting and research needs. A joint statement of the European Association for the Study of Diabetes and the American Diabetes Association diabetes technology working group. *Diabetologia, 58*(5), 862–870.

Howes, D. (2005). Architecture of the senses. In M. Zardini (Ed.), *Sense of the city: An alternate approach to urbanism* (pp. 322–331). CCA: Montreal.

International Diabetes Federation. (2015). *IDF Diabetes Atlas* (7th ed.). Brussels, Belgium: International Diabetes Federation. http://www.diabetes-atlas.org.

Jackson, M. (2002). Familiar and foreign bodies: A phenomenological exploration of the human-technology interface. *Journal of the Royal Anthropological Institute, 8*(2), 333–346.

Latour, B. (1993). *We have never been modern.* London: Prentice Hall.

Leder, D. (1990). *The absent body.* Chicago: University of Chicago Press.

Merleau-Ponty, M., & Edie, J. M. (1964). *the primacy of perception: and other essays on phenomenological psychology, the philosophy of art, history and politics.* Evanston, Il: Northwestern University Press.

Miller, D. (2001). *Consumption: Theory and issues in the study of consumption.* London: Routledge.

Mol, A. (2002). *The body multiple: Ontology in medical practice.* Durham, NC: Duke University Press.

Mol, A., & Law, J. (2004). Embodied action, enacted bodies: The example of hypoglycaemia. *Body and Society, 10*(2–3), 43–62.

NICE. (2008). *Diabetes (type 1) insulin pump therapy guidance.* TA57. London: National Institute for Clinical Excellence.

Norris, L. (2004). Shedding skins the materiality of divestment in India. *Journal of Material Culture, 9*(1), 59–71.

Pickup, J., Keen, H., Viberti, G., & Bilous, R. (1981). Patient reactions to long-term outpatient treatment with continuous subcutaneous insulin infusion. *British medical journal (Clinical research ed.), 282*(6266), 766–768.

Scheldemen, G. (2010). Technokids? Insulin pumps incorporated in young people's bodies and lives. In J. Edwards, P. Harvey, & P. Wade (Eds.),

Technologized images (pp. 137–159). Berghahn Series: Technologized Bodies.

Strathern, M. (1988). *The gender of the gift: Problems with women and problems with society in Melanesia.* Oakland, CA: University of California.

Seltin, J. (2009). Production of the post-human: Political economies of bodies and technology. *Parrhesia, 8,* 43–59.

Taylor, J. (2005). Surfacing the body interior. *Annual Review of Anthropology, 34,* 741–756.

Willerslev, R. (2007). To have the world at a distance: Reconsidering the significance of vision for social anthropology. In C. Grasseni (Ed.), *Skilled visions: Between apprencticeship and standards* (pp. 23–46). Oxford: Berghahn.

Woolgar, S. and Lazaun, J. (2013). The wrong Bin Bag: A turn to ontology in science and technology studies? *Social Studies of Science, 43,* pp. 321–340.

5

Redrawing Boundaries Around the Self: The Case of Self-Quantifying Technologies

Farzana Dudhwala

Introduction

Over the past decade or so, there has been a significant change in the way people are using technologies on themselves and for themselves. The formation of the group known as the 'Quantified Self' in 2007 marked the beginning of a new era of consumer wearables and technologies, and characterised a surge in the innovation and marketing of devices which claim to monitor, track, record, measure, and quantify the self. Heart rate, steps, calories, mood, blood glucose levels, sleep, and weight are just some examples of the many aspects of the self that can be quantified. This is not to say that the market has been fuelled solely by members of the Quantified Self group, but rather that the

---

All interview material used in this chapter was gained with informed consent and is used with permission.

F. Dudhwala (✉)
Nuffield Department of Primary Care Health Sciences,
University of Oxford, Oxford, UK
e-mail: farzana.dudhwala@phc.ox.ac.uk

© The Author(s) 2018
R. Lynch and C. Farrington (eds.), *Quantified Lives and Vital Data*,
Health, Technology and Society, https://doi.org/10.1057/978-1-349-95235-9_5

formation of the group symbolised the crystallisation of a new kind of interest in the 'self', piqued by the capabilities of technologies that are increasingly accessible to the general public rather than being confined to a select few experts.

Access to blood glucose levels, for instance, was largely the preserve of medical experts, or at best, those with diabetes. Similarly, being able to access one's own heart rate over a prolonged period of time was often only possible in a hospital and when attached to a machine of sorts. And detailed knowledge of one's own sleep patterns was only available by going to a sleep laboratory and having electrodes attached to the head. Now technologies are readily available and accessible such that anyone with some disposable income can buy them and have access to these things for themselves. And people are doing them: people are using these technologies to get a better sense of their 'health', their 'mood', their 'fitness' and their 'behaviour'—people are using these technologies to get a better sense of their 'self'.

These personal medical devices, or 'self-quantifying technologies' as they will be referred to more generally in this chapter, are driving subtle changes in the way that care of the self is done. Increasingly, these technologies are not only being used by people who are suffering from an illness (although some undoubtedly will be), but by those who are curious to know more about themselves, who want to improve some aspect of their health or who are trying to maintain a certain level of wellness (e.g. Swan 2009; Lupton 2013).

Given that these technologies have made it much more possible to engage in activities which apparently give a better sense of 'self', it is pertinent to question precisely what the role of these technologies is and how they might warrant a shift in how we conceive of the very notion of 'self'. This chapter thus explores how, in practice, boundaries are made around the self in the context of self-quantification, asking questions such as: what does or does not get included in the 'self'? What role do these technologies have in the making/doing of the 'self'? To what extent does it make sense to continue to talk about knowledge of the 'self' as a singular and fixed entity rather than talking about the ways in which interaction/intra-action with these self-quantifying technologies fosters a constant enactment of fluid and multiple 'selves'?

Taking empirical insights from a 4-year multi-sited ethnography of the 'Quantified Self' group, I discuss issues of agency and performativity using science and technology studies (henceforth 'STS') sensibilities to investigate how boundaries are made around the self using self-quantifying technologies. The chapter begins by introducing the 'Quantified Self' and explaining why it is a privileged case from which to study the issues discussed above. I then offer some empirical material, in the form of vignettes, drawn from interviews conducted with members of the Quantified Self to address issues of boundary making and the doing of the self. The vignettes raise issues regarding the performative nature of self-quantifying technologies, and therefore, in the next part of the chapter, I discuss matters of agency and performativity to help to explain the relationship between these self-quantifying technologies and the self.

Many of the existing theories of agency and performativity do not go far enough in questioning the ontological nature of the entities that they purport to explain, and I therefore suggest an engagement with Karen Barad's theory of 'agential realism' as a way to overcome some of these shortcomings. Following a short foray into the quantum experiments that underpin Barad's ideas, I assess the usefulness of her concepts of 'intra-action' and 'agential cutting' for understanding how new boundaries around the self are being drawn and constantly redrawn through the use of self-quantifying technologies, resulting in the production of fluid and multiple selves.

The 'Quantified Self'

The 'Quantified Self' ('QS' for short) is a self-proclaimed 'collaboration of users and tool makers' founded by Gary Wolf and Kevin Kelly in 2007 (Wolf 2011). There are over 80,000 members of the Quantified Self dispersed throughout the world, with more than 100 cities hosting their own QS 'Meetup'. Meetups are meetings that are organised every one or two months and consist of a series of presentations by group members about their self-quantifying behaviours. Typically, the presentations are structured around the following three questions: 'What I did', 'How I did it' and 'What I learned'. The presentations are often accompanied by a slide show depicting visualisations of what has been quantified and are followed by questions from group members in the audience. The discussions then continue in a nearby pub, where presenters and audience members talk some more about self-quantification practices and generally catch up over a drink.

For 4 years, I attended these Meetups (primarily in London, but also several in Manchester, Oxford, Amsterdam and San Francisco), joined in with the post-Meetup pub discussions, interviewed 35 members of the Quantified Self, watched 40 videos of presentations given at the Meetups and followed the Quantified Self web forum where people ask questions and discuss self-quantification practices. The empirical material in this chapter comes directly from this 4-year multi-sited ethnography.

People who participate in, and are members of, the QS are from all walks of life. I have interviewed and talked to entrepreneurs, teachers, consultants, homemakers, academics, doctors, lawyers, engineers, students, and office workers. Some of them may have chronic conditions such as diabetes or high blood pressure, but the majority of the members of the QS are those simply with a curiosity about themselves. They also have the ability and willingness to use self-quantifying technologies to monitor, track, measure or record some aspect of themselves or their behaviour for the purposes of increasing self-knowledge. In terms of the gender make-up of the group, whilst the number of women participating in the QS is increasing, this is still somewhat a male-dominated area.

Self-quantification via the use of digital technologies that are personal and portable is different from self-quantification via the use of non-digital technologies like paper-based diaries, or from fixed hospital machines. The digital nature of the technologies means that the amount of data that can be collected has increased exponentially. Moreover, the resultant data can be analysed in much more sophisticated and complex ways with the help of computing power.

Whilst there are no shortages of machines that can track selves and bodies in hospitals, there is something very different about the use of personal, portable technologies that are operated by self-quantifiers *for* themselves, rather than *on* them by an expert. In the former case, patients can be seen as the passive recipients of the expert's analysis and interpretation about what the technology is showing. In the latter case, people are seemingly accountable for their own self-quantification. They are accountable for the collection of their data and consequent analysis. That is not to say that there are no other entities involved in this process, but there is a very apparent shift in the locus of accountability from expert to self.

The Quantified Self group is an ideal case from which to understand how the self is 'done' through the use of self-quantifying technologies. In her ethnographic study of the production of scientific knowledge, Hélène Mialet (2012, p. 191) uses Stephen Hawking as the sole case study from which to draw conclusions that are applied much more generally. The reason for doing so, she argues, is that the extreme case of Hawking's disability allows her to highlight the very processes that are often ubiquitous in the making of knowledge, yet are hidden from view. I make a similar argument for the choice of using the Quantified Self as the case study for this research. Whilst they might be seen as an extreme example of self-quantification with no further application beyond their own case, I argue that it is the very directed way in which they navigate the self through the use of these self-quantifying technologies that highlight the processes by which self-measuring devices in general come to play a part in the production of a certain 'self' in specific contexts. The vignettes below begin to illustrate this point.

Practices of Self-quantification 1

Guessing Glucose Levels

Ben is a member of the London Quantified Self group who (at the time of this research) was in his early thirties and a keen runner. He was recently diagnosed as having type 1 diabetes—a condition where the pancreas does not produce any insulin (the hormone responsible for regulating the amount of glucose in the blood). For someone who is a keen athlete, this diagnosis was a big blow, who told me that he worried he would not be able to keep up with his running.

He used to go for runs without self-tracking or taking a watch and described himself as a 'happy-go-lucky kind of guy'. Since the diagnosis, however, Ben acquired a blood glucose monitor and measured his blood glucose level several times a day, and also started to use watches and apps on his mobile phone to track his runs.

During the hour that we spoke, Ben took out his blood glucose monitor and told me that he would guess what his blood glucose level was, whilst simultaneously measuring it with his device to see if he could guess it. When telling me how many millimoles per litre (mmol/L) of glucose he thought he had in his blood at that moment, he started to describe his day to me.

He explained that he had drunk one cup of coffee and that he thought that the lunch he had eaten a couple of hours earlier was quite low in carbohydrates. He also told me that he had rushed to meet me as he was running a little late. Taking all this into account, he guessed that his blood glucose level would be about 6.5 mmol/L (he is usually somewhere between 4 and 8 mmol/L).

He then took out an instrument which he used to prick his finger. He guided the resultant droplet of blood to a strip on the bottom of the device. The display was facing me, and so I was the first to see the blood glucose level indicated on the screen. It showed 7.5 mmol/L.

Relative to where he told me he normally was, this was evidently quite a high reading. As he turned the device so that he too could see the reading, he looked a little surprised. He smiled and immediately started to justify why his reading was much higher than he thought it was: the low-carb lunch he ate was in a coffee shop, and therefore, it was difficult to tell how much extra sugar they put into the food to make it taste better; the coffee he had was in a larger mug than usual; and his walk may not have been as brisk as he thought it was.

Overruling the Recommended 'Recovery Time'

I had known Leo as a QS member from London for at least 2 years—he was one of the first people I met at my first QS Meetup there. Leo told me that without knowing the name 'The Quantified Self' he had already been tracking himself for many years, accumulating over 8 years' worth of weight data. He said that he would also describe himself as a 'gadget lover' and that he had a disposable income which allowed him to buy and try out a number of different devices. The latest device he had bought was a Garmin sports watch—a running watch that measures speed, distance and route of the run by using the in-built GPS chip, as well as heart rate by connecting to a chest strap.

Leo was pretty excited about this new watch—he told me that it was the best he'd ever had. One of the most exciting features of this watch for Leo was that at the end of a run, the watch gave an estimate for how long he should wait to recover before going on his next run. In general, Leo said that his watch would tell him to wait between 6 and 36 h between runs, which he thought was reasonable. A few days ago, however, it told him to wait a significantly longer time. 'I ran six and a half miles—which is not a lot for me—just a week ago, and it said to sit down and rest for three days. Like, *THREE DAYS?* I'm like, what? But the thing is that actually the watch had said that, and it did coincide with how I felt. I was just wiped. Like I was totally missing a gear'. I asked him whether he actually waited the recommended three days before going on his next run, and he admitted that he had been for a run only two days after.

I asked him why he disregarded the advice given to him by his watch. He reasoned that 'I use the watch as a rough guide—what I'm trying to do right now is gauge it against my mental feelings—does the reading fit with how I feel? And so far it's been pretty good—and so as I start to trust it more as a guide, I might give it more weighting—but I'll never probably give it absolute weighting—and what it's not saying is that for the next 3 days stay at home, don't go out, don't go to work, just that I should take it easy…' In other words, he told me that the watch was best used as a heuristic rather than treated as gospel.

Two Differing Responses

These vignettes depict two practices of self-quantification. In the first, we encounter Ben, a recently diagnosed diabetic who went from being a 'happy-go-lucky' guy who didn't measure or track his runs to now using a blood glucose monitor several times a day as well as using an app to track his runs. In the second vignette, we meet Leo, a keen self-quantifier who says he has been tracking himself since before the 'Quantified Self' was formed as an established group. In both instances, a technology is used to quantify some aspect of the self (blood glucose levels for Ben and running activity for Leo), and some output is received (mmol/L of glucose in blood and running metrics coupled with estimated rest period).

Interestingly, the consequent reactions to the outputs of the technology were very different in both cases. For Ben, when the blood glucose monitor revealed that his blood glucose level was particularly high relative to his normal range, and higher than his own guess about what it was, his narrative account of his day rapidly changed. He felt the need to justify why it could have been the case that his meal may have contained more sugar than he thought, or how his walk may not have been as brisk as he had originally indicated, and so on. Of course, there was nothing stopping him from sticking to his original narrative, but it seemed as though the reading on the device made his original assertions less credible to himself, or at the very least compelled him to revise certain aspects of his narrative. In a sense, Ben felt the need to justify himself so that his explanation of events and the reading on the device corroborated each other.

This has some parallels with Festinger's (1957) concept of 'cognitive dissonance'—the term used to describe the stress or anxiety felt by someone who holds two or more contradictory beliefs at once, or when some information is discovered which opposes a pre-existing belief. In this case, the blood glucose monitor opposed the narrative account that Ben had described to me, and which had led to the belief or feeling that his blood glucose level was much lower than the monitor showed.

Perhaps 'technological dissonance' might be a more apt term to use here—where the self-quantifying technology has given some information or data that contradicts what one feels or thinks one knows about oneself, causing feelings of anxiety or uncertainty.

The reading on Leo's device, however, led to a different type of reaction. He looked at the reading on the watch and disregarded the advice that it gave him to rest for three days. For Leo, the watch was more of a rough guide to be used to check in with how he was feeling and then decide how much weighting to give to the advice. He even admitted that he felt as though he was 'totally missing a gear', yet this was not enough for him to have taken the recommended three days off from running. So why in one instance of self-quantification did Ben listen to what the self-quantifying technology told him, whereas in the other instance Leo ignored it?

There are a number of possible explanations. One is that Leo has less trust in the self-quantifying technologies and therefore only uses them as a heuristic rather than as something by which he ought to be commanded. But this explanation is somewhat unsatisfactory—Leo is a self-proclaimed gadget lover and he had been heavily praising this Garmin Watch as one of the best he has had. It seems unlikely that the reason is to do with scepticism of the technology. Another explanation could be that the *kind* of information that is given by two devices is different, and that this could be causing the differences in response.

The blood glucose monitor used by Ben tests the chemicals of the blood to produce a measure of how much glucose is present—if this level is too high or too low, it risks hypoglycaemia or hyperglycaemia, which could prove fatal. This is different to a chest strap monitoring the user's heart rate and telling them to rest for a few days. Although there is a possibility that the user may get injured from over-training, the consequences seem much more severe in the former case than in the latter. Is there something, then, about the *type* of measurement that indicates to what extent the output of a self-quantification may lead to action or not? Two further practices of self-quantification will help to unpick this question.

Practices of Self-quantification 2

Not Enough Calories Burned

Tamara had generously given up time on her lunch break to meet with me near her offices in Soho in London. She worked for a social media company and had recently become interested in self-quantification. Alongside tracking her finances through readily available data from her debit card expenditure and Oyster card usage (a contactless prepaid card used for public transport in London), she had recently downloaded the 'Map My Ride' app on her mobile phone. This app is designed for cyclists and measures and records the distance cycled, speed travelled, location/route, and calories burned during the ride.

Tamara cycled to work every day. For a long time, she felt as though her ride to work required substantial effort and she commended herself for choosing to cycle rather than taking public transport each day. When she got into work, Tamara would routinely grab a cup of coffee from the kitchen, along with a morning snack—often a croissant or a pastry—which she consumed happily without guilt since she had cycled into work in the morning and thought she had earned a treat.

As her curiosity increased with her newfound interest in self-quantification, Tamara begun to track her commute to work with the Map My Ride app. After seeing the post-ride data on her app, Tamara told me that being able to see the number of calories burned with each ride actually made her feel worse. She told me that she had previously felt good about her rides, but when she saw that she had barely burned any calories in relation to the amount of effort she had perceived herself exerting, it was disappointing.

Furthermore, her feeling of disappointment was made even worse when she started to use the 'food logging' feature of the app—which allows the user to input the food they consume to be told an estimate of the amount of calories in the food. Comparing the number of calories burned in her morning cycle to the number of calories in a croissant/pastry alerted her to the fact that the morning cycle 'did not justify' her being able to enjoy her morning snack.

An Improved Vo2 Max

Samuel was one of the oldest people that I had come across who was involved in practices of self-quantification. At the time that we met for over two and half hours in the dining area of the Marriott Hotel at King's Cross Station in London, Samuel was 72 years old. One of the first things he told me was that he had become interested in preventative health in 2006, and he spent a lot of time wondering how he could live longer and in good health. His aim was to 'get to a hundred, be physically fit, mentally fit, sexually fit, and actively contribute in all sorts of ways'.

Samuel told me that he became concerned when, 8 years previously, he had begun to present with symptoms that indicated early ageing: he had high blood pressure and was overweight. Since then, he started running experiments on himself to understand the lifestyle and diet factors that might reverse these signs of ageing and contribute to longevity. He started to take supplements, restricted his calorie intake and exercised much more rigorously. He proudly proclaimed that he lost 22 kg during this time and managed to reduce his blood pressure. He also said that he had more energy now than ever, and that he felt physically and mentally like a 30-year-old.

For Samuel, even more impressive than his weight loss and reduced blood pressure were the gains he saw in his fitness levels, which he assessed primarily by looking at his Vo2 max. (Vo2 max is a measure of the maximum volume of oxygen that a person can use, measured in millilitres per kg of body weight per minute—the higher the Vo2 max value, the more intensely the person can exercise). When he first measured his Vo2 max level, it was 23 ml/kg/min. He told me at this point that a young athlete would have a Vo2 max in the region of 60 ml/kg/min or more.

Alongside taking more care of his diet and exercise regime, Samuel also bought a device which would 'train' the muscles that allowed him to breathe to be stronger and more efficient. Quite simply, it was a device that he had to breathe into through various levels of resistance to increase the amount of oxygen he could take in with each breath.

After a few years of his new regime of supplements, diet, exercise and breathing training, Samuel increased his Vo2 max to over 30 ml/kg/min—something he told me that he was very proud of.

The Effect of Different Types of Measurement

Here we have two more self-quantification practices: the first depicting someone who began to track her commute into work each day and the second depicting someone experimenting on himself to increase longevity and health. The experience of Tamara's bicycle ride into work raises some important questions about the role of technology in the 'making' or 'doing' of the self. Before Tamara looked at the data on her MapMyRide app, her experience of the ride was very different in comparison with her experience after she looked at it. Before looking at the data on the app, she viewed her ride as positive, but when looking at the data on her app her experience of her ride became less so. Her ride *without* the app was experienced much more positively than her ride *with* the app.

One of the achievements of Samuel's self-quantification practices is increasing his Vo2 max from 23 ml/kg/min to over 30 ml/kg/min. This highlights that it is much more fruitful to consider the practice of self-quantification as being productive rather than representative. In one sense, it could be argued that it is easier to judge feeling good about a particular bike ride (the rider may have felt particularly fast, strong, fit, exerted or 'worked out'), than it is to 'feel' a 7 ml/kg/min increase in Vo2 max. In this sense, the technologies used to measure Vo2 max are a fundamental part of the Vo2 max, since without it Samuel has very little, if any, indicator of a 7 ml/kg/min increase.

The technology practices therefore seem to have an important bearing on Samuel as a self that has an increased Vo2 max, and therefore a self who is succeeding on his quest for longevity and good health. Perhaps these technology practices can even be said to *perform* this aspect of Samuel. What might it mean to argue that the practice of self-quantification is 'performative'?

The Performative Nature of Self-Quantification

There are many variations and interpretations of 'performativity' in the literature. Often, the notion of performativity is thought of in the context of questions such as 'can saying make it so?' (Austin 1962, p. 7). Austin (1962, p. 12) argued that there are 'some cases…in which to say something is to do something; or in which by saying or in saying something we are doing something'. For example, Austin maintains that uttering the words 'I do' at a wedding is actively performing something in that moment: it is performing the marriage of the two people who say them. However, speech acts are not the only instances where performativity is important. Others have appropriated their own definitions of the concept in a number of different domains.

Goffman's (1959) notion of performativity, for example, involves distinguishing between a frontstage and a backstage 'performance' of the self, by the self. The latter is thought to be the 'true' self, whereas the former is the 'performance' or the role played according to social conventions and norms. This notion of performativity is based on a literal dramaturgical reading of the term, using metaphors from theatre to explain its workings. However, the performativity that I am concerned with focuses on the more recent instantiations of the term, which move away from the dramaturgical/representational aspect and into the ontological sphere.

Butler (1993, 2010, 2013), for instance, clearly distinguishes her notion of performativity from Goffman's. For Goffman, the self has a stable interiority (the 'backstage' self) and the performance is a set of external roles played by this self with regard to social norms and expectations. For Butler, however, there is no stable interior 'self' (Butler 2013). In fact, the very idea of interiority is itself performed and regulated. This means that the fact that something appears to be a given or seen as a pre-existing interiority is precisely the result of it being repeatedly performed and reified as such. Therefore, to say that something is performatively constituted is to say that it does not have a stable core prior to the behaviours and expressions that bring it into being.

However, to maintain something as an interiority in the way that Butler outlines, there is a sense in which, as Law and Singleton (2000) argue, performances must rely on previous performances—either to repeat/reify them or perhaps to modify them and suggest alternatives. How are these performances (or performances of previous performances) done? Law and Singleton's version of performativity rests upon the assumption of a number of heterogeneous elements which 'assemble' together to produce certain consequences (the performance).

In the context of self-quantification, this would mean an assemblage of entities such as, in the case of Ben, the blood glucose monitor, sugar, blood, food, fingers and a 'normal' range of mmol/L. The coming together of these entities, at least according to Law and Singleton's ideas, performs Ben's state of having a higher blood sugar level than both what he had intuited and relative to his normal range. However, this analysis of the practice of self-quantification still leaves too many questions unanswered. Why these specific entities? How do they come together? Why was the coffee table at which Ben and I were sitting not relevant, or the lighting in the cafe, or the colour of my jumper? In other words, it could be otherwise (c.f. Woolgar 2014)! Further, could it be that we have jumped the gun in assuming that the 'entities' exist in and of themselves in that particular form—what performances had to be performed to get to a 'blood glucose monitor' in the first place, for example? The problem with Law and Singleton's version of performativity, therefore, is first that it doesn't account for how particular entities are 'chosen' for assemblage, and second, it is implied that these heterogeneous entities pre-exist the attempts to assemble them—that they are the cause for some consequential action.

From a Baradian reading of performance, these heterogeneous assemblages are not a 'given'. They are not pre-existing jigsaw shapes just waiting to be put together. This is similar to Butler's (2013) argument that there is no pre-existing stable core to gender. However, the two theorists depart on their conceptions of what 'matters'. Butler relies heavily, if not solely, on discursive practices as performing all else, neglecting to engage with the role of materiality. For Barad, discursive practices are only one part of performativity, and both matter and discourse are invoked in a performance at the same time.

For Barad, everything/anything has the *potential* for agency. She argues that it makes no sense to assume that there is a distinction between human and material agency because that would presume that either had certain qualities about them which preceded interaction with them. For Barad, 'there are no such independently existing objects with inherent characteristics' (2003, p. 816). For this reason, Barad argues that the representationalist account of the world, where, for example, scientists purport to merely *represent* the reality that is already out there, cannot hold. Barad describes her way of looking at the world as an 'agential realist ontology' and arrives at this theory through the use of a 'diffractive methodology' in which she uses the insights of quantum physics to think about the nature of the world. Her theory is largely rooted in the infamous debates surrounding the 'double-slit experiments' in quantum physics between Albert Einstein and Niels Bohr (Einstein et al. 1935; Bohr 1935).

A Short Foray into Quantum Mechanics: The Double-Slit Experiments

The double-slit experiment was designed to determine whether a given entity exhibits a 'particle-like' pattern or a 'wave-like' pattern when passing through a piece of apparatus with two slits in it. The experiment was designed so that the projection of the entity that is fired through it can be seen on a screen. If the entity is a particle, then it can only enter through one of the two slits and the projection on the screen will be directly opposite the slit that it passed through. This is because the nature of a particle is such that it can only occupy a certain space at a certain time—it cannot be in two places at once. If, however, the entity is wave-like, then it is not bound by space and time since it travels in such a way that it can occupy a greater space through time. Therefore, the projection will reveal an overlapping concentric wave-like pattern.

When doing this experiment with an electron, one would expect (given the commonly held view that an electron is a particle rather than a wave) that the projections would be in two discreet places opposite the two slits. However, the experiments actually resulted in a projection that showed an overlapping concentric wave pattern. To understand how this was possible, Einstein devised an experiment to observe which slit the particles went through. He put a spring on one of the slits which would account for movement if the entity went through it. Einstein argued that if it went through just one slit (like a particle) but had a diffraction/wave pattern (like a wave), then an inherent contradiction in quantum physics would be unearthed and we would therefore need a new way to think about how to explain the entities in the world.

However, Bohr (the physicist at the heart of Barad's work) argued that Einstein was mistaken in his assumptions. Bohr argued that in adding the spring, Einstein changed the *apparatus* that was fundamental in the production of both the entity and its projection. In other words, he argued that the results of any experiment are the entanglement of the apparatus used and the observed object. In effect, 'the very nature of the entity—its ontology—changes (or rather becomes differently determinate) depending on the experimental apparatus used to determine its nature' (Barad 2012, p. 42). This interpretation of events has since become known as the 'Copenhagen Interpretation'.

Heisenberg was dissatisfied with Bohr's interpretation and argued that the reason that the pattern changes from a wave to a particle pattern is because the change made to the apparatus is intervening in the experiment and thus disturbing the entity. This, he argued, constrains what we can know about the entity, because each measurement disturbs what it is that is being measured—so trying to measure the disturbance includes within it its own disturbance and so on. Since it would always be uncertain what the precise disturbance was, he called this the 'uncertainty principle'.

Yet again, Bohr was unconvinced. He argued that Heisenberg wrongly characterised the events as being to do with uncertainty. Instead, Bohr argued that the issue was one of 'determinacy'. When we make a measurement, he maintained, it is not that we disturb the 'true thing' that is being measured and so that our knowledge is consequently uncertain with regard to the 'objective truth'. It is that *there are no such 'true things' to begin with*. There is no measurement-independent 'stuff' waiting for the right experiment to uncover it. The interaction of the apparatuses and the conditions of the experiment *are* the things-in-being. They do not exist outside of this.

These quantum entanglements have been discussed here not because of their potential impact on scientific thinking, but rather because of the important philosophical implications of the debates and the various justifications. And it is the philosophical implications of Bohr's account in particular that are the most useful for us, since he effectively reconceptualised the ontological nature of the world in his explanations of what was going on in the double-slit experiments.

For Bohr, the real issue was that things are 'indeterminate': there are no things before the measurement and it is the very act of measurement that produces determinate boundaries. So, whilst Heisenberg was dealing with what he considered to be an *epistemological* problem—that of *how* to know things—Bohr was working with an *ontological* problem, of *what* it is we are trying to know in the first place.

Following this, Barad maintains that there is no world already 'out there', and it is *made* or only *becomes* in the moment where 'intra-action' occurs: 'the world is intra-activity in its differential mattering' (Barad 2003, p. 817). 'Intra-action' is a term used to refer to a simultaneously reciprocal action between different entities, and it is only in these moments that specific things may become apparent. These constantly ongoing intra-actions are termed 'material-discursive practices', and it is through these practices that certain boundaries are enacted and performed.

This world view has certain implications for both STS and an analysis of the role of self-quantifying technologies in creating boundaries around the self. Subscribing to an agential realist ontology would lead to the view that a given phenomenon is not the 'result' of experiments or research. The experiments or the research process *is/becomes* the phenomenon itself. That is, they play a crucial role in its constitution as a phenomenon, which only becomes *that* phenomenon with *those* particular experiments or research process. What does this mean for the role of self-quantifying technologies in the production of a quantified self? To what extent does the very act of self-quantification produce a boundary around the self, and in turn perform the self?

Let us think about this in relation to the vignettes above. Tamara's ride into work was a different thing altogether when she quantified it. Before the addition of the MapMyRun app, the bike ride was an effortful ride which justified the eating of a croissant. After it had been quantified using the app, however, it became a disappointing ride which failed to meet expectations regarding calories burned vis-a-vis perceived effort. The whole phenomenon was a different entity altogether.

Similarly, we can in some respects see how, at least for Ben, the use of the blood glucose monitor *produces* a certain type of self rather than merely describing it. Prior to measuring his blood glucose level with the monitor, we could say that he was 'Ben-with-relatively-normal-blood-glucose-levels', or 'Ben-who-can-intuit-his-own-blood-glucose-level' or 'Ben-who-is-self-aware'. However, the use of the monitor shifts this somewhat. With the reading on the device, he becomes 'Ben-with-relatively-high-blood-glucose-levels' or 'Ben-who-is-unaware-of-his-own-blood-glucose-levels' or 'Ben-who-is-not-self-aware', for example. But how are certain aspects decided as being *the* relevant ones if there exist a number of potential other aspects that could be focused on? Once again, it seems as though 'it could be otherwise', yet how does one decide amongst these potential others? Is this even possible?

In the next part of this chapter, I discuss intra-action with regard to the self. In particular, I discuss how the notion of 'agential cutting' is a useful way in which to understand how boundaries are made around the self, and potentially explain how certain 'otherwises' are chosen over others.

Self-Intra-Action

Whilst the theory of agential realism does not explicitly focus on the 'self', Barad's 'On Touching—The Inhuman That Therefore I Am' (2013) describes the discovery of the electron in the nineteenth century and then uses this to question the very notion of the 'self'. Her ideas about the self have important implications for thinking about the concept of the 'agential self' in the context of using self-quantifying technologies.

For many, the perception of touch involves some sort of 'contact' (fingers touching one another or the touch/contact involved in holding a pen). A scientific explanation of touching, however, turns that notion on its head. Barad (2013) explains that when 'touching' something, you are never really *in contact* with that thing. In fact, the electrons in the atoms of your fingers are actually electromagnetically *repulsing* the electrons in the atoms of the pen. The electrons can never, and will never, come into direct contact with one another—it is physically impossible. This allows Barad provocatively to assert that 'repulsion is at the core of attraction' (2013, p. 209).

What does this have to do with the nature of the self? Physically, the electron is a 'single point carrying a negative charge'. Since the electron is a point particle and therefore cannot have a radius (it is zero dimensional), then its interaction with its surroundings is infinite. Further, these surroundings are created by its own electromagnetic field through the exchange of a virtual photon with itself, and so its interaction with itself is also infinite. This also makes it very difficult to trace the separation between the electron and its own self-created environment. (In quantum physics, this environment is known as the 'void' and the electron is the 'particle'.)

Since the interaction of the electron with its surroundings is theoretically infinite (physicists refer to this as 'an infinite sum over all possibilities'), and the electron, in creating and then absorbing its own photon, is intra-acting with itself, it follows that the possibilities for self-intra-action in general are also infinite. As Barad (2013, p. 213) argues, 'self-touching is an encounter with the alterity of the self. Matter is an enfolding, an involution, it cannot help touching itself, and in this self-touching it comes into contact with the infinite alterity that it is'.

So, for Barad, the self intra-acts with itself and this *self-intra-action* indicates that the very notion of identity can be challenged. What, then, is the 'self' according to Barad's argument? If, as she tells us, the quantum of an electromagnetic field is a photon, and the quantum of a gravitational field is a graviton, then what is the quantum of the self? Is the comparison even possible? This is a question that Barad is puzzled by too. Through her work on amoeba colonies (slime moulds which seamlessly morph from single-cell organisms into aggregate complex organisms with their own immune and nervous systems), she questions the very definition of what counts and what does not count as an 'individual' (Barad 2012). Are the amoeba colonies an aggregate of individuals or do they become one single entity? In the same vein, is the self an aggregate of, for example, individual emotions, chemical responses, self-quantifying technologies and negative charges which never actually come into contact, or is it a single and cohesive entity?

If the former, then the 'self' is a perversion simply in its 'being' since it is the aggregate of many individual selves touching or intra-acting with themselves. The self here both projects and envelops itself at the same time. Self-quantifying technologies, therefore, are at once with*out* and with*in* the self. They are *without* in the sense that these are 'external' technologies quantifying the self and indicating to it what that self is. However, they are also *within* in the sense that it is the self that is using the technologies to quantify itself and interpret what it is being told. Therefore, the self is simultaneously 'being done to' and 'doing' in the same way that the electron is absorbing the very photon that it itself emits.

Although the case of the electron as described by Barad contains the possibility for an infinite number of potentialities and alterities, she does not fully explain why one particular potentiality comes into being rather than another. *That* intra-action happens is explained in great detail by Barad—but why it happens in any one particular formulation over another is less clear. The concept of 'agential cutting' is Barad's attempt to address this problem.

Boundary Making Through Agential Cutting

The notion of an *agential cut* is an intriguing aspect of Barad's theory of *Agential Realism*, especially with regard to understanding the self. An *agential cut* is the temporary separation of certain phenomena. That is, agential cutting is the making of a temporary boundary between phenomena so that they can be studied, communicated, enacted or understood. An *agential cut* momentarily defocuses everything except for the phenomenon in question. Without these *agential cuts*, everything is enmeshed in an intertwined web of relational ontology where nothing can be differentiated from, or conceived of, without anything else. Thus, according to Barad, making an *agential cut* allows certain phenomena to be momentarily distinguished and performed.

Barad also argues that 'agential cuts do not mark some absolute separation but a cutting together/apart—a "holding together" of the disparate itself' (Barad 2012, p. 46). So as well as defocusing some things, it brings and holds together others. The *agential cut* can thus be seen as the making of a boundary, which requires a separation of some things to enact the holding together of others.

According to this idea, when sharing 'knowledge' about something, we are sharing with others the specific *agential cut* that we have made involving particular *apparatuses* and *discourse*. In the context of people using self-quantifying technologies, how are agential cuts made when drawing a boundary around what the 'self' encompasses? Is it possible to know other peoples' agential cuts—to know what they have separated and what they are trying to hold together?

The self that concerns this research is the self that is quantified using some sort of self-quantifying technology. That is the crucial element in what does, and what does not, get included in the agential cut, or to put it more broadly, in the boundary around the self. What then counts as a 'self-quantifying technology' to the people that are using it? Working backwards from Barad's notion of agential cutting, we find that agential cutting is the result of an intra-action, which itself is the production of the inextricable coming together of what she terms 'discourse' and 'apparatus'.

Very briefly, discourse is not simply a word used to describe what is said, but also that which enables or restricts what *can* be said. Apparatuses are not simply laboratory tools or even self-quantifying technologies that are used to uncover the 'truth' or find out the 'real' results. For Barad, 'apparatuses produce differences that matter—they are boundary making practices that are formative of matter and meaning, productive of, and part of, the phenomena produced' (Barad 2007, p. 146). Thus, the apparatus and the phenomena cannot be separated.

This idea can be linked back to Bohr's criticism of Einstein's idea to add a spring to the double-slit experiment to observe or measure what was going on. Bohr's main objection to changing the apparatus of the experiment (by adding something to it) was that it would be measuring and producing an entirely different phenomenon altogether. It could no longer be said to be the same thing.

If we return to the vignettes presented at the beginning of this chapter, what might count as the self-quantifying technology in each of them, and why? In the case of Tamara (as with all the vignettes), there is a seemingly obvious answer to the question of what the self-quantifying technology is for her—the MapMyRun app—not least because it is the very focus of the conversation that I had with her about self-quantification. But why is this the case? There are many things involved in her commute to work: the bicycle, traffic lights, her helmet, etc. Why were these things not taken to be the self-quantifying technologies? Perhaps, self-quantifying technologies in this instance ought to be something that produces a difference that matters.

In Tamara's case, we can reasonably assume that the only thing that significantly changed in those two instances was the use of the MapMyRide app—she had the same bicycle, we can assume that the traffic lights had not changed, and she wore the same helmet. Thus, the app can be considered to be the relevant self-quantifying technology. Similarly, Ben's blood glucose monitor was complicit in producing a difference that mattered. In fact, the reading on the machine was the reason that he changed his entire narrative about his day.

The distinction between the concepts of *discourse* and *apparatus* can be quite confusing since they are both, by Barad's own theory, upshots of some agential cut, rather than independently existing entities. The distinction between them is therefore rather contrived—and the examples from the vignettes above show that in each case, the self-quantifying technologies can be read as both apparatus and discourse interchangeably. However, in a more general sense, the concepts of *discourse* and *apparatus* allow us to move beyond questions rooted in naïve representationalism, such as 'are these technologies accurate enough to tell us who/what we really are?', to more pertinent questions rooted in ideas of performativity, such as 'to what extent are these self-quantifying technologies implicated in the 'doing' of the self?'.

They are, therefore, also useful in understanding the implications of self-quantifying technologies on agency and performativity, and in trying to ascertain what might count as a self-quantifying technology in the first place. The two main ideas behind the concepts of *discourse* and *apparatus* in this context are firstly that they enable/constrain what can/cannot be said, and secondly, they produce 'differences that matter'. From my interviews and observations, it is apparent that perhaps one of the most important aspects of self-quantifying technologies are that they enable (and also have the capacity to constrain) what can and cannot be said. The blood monitor enabled Ben to say that he has diabetes and a high blood sugar level at the moment, but also constrained him in the sense that he felt that he needed to change the original narrative that he gave about his day. Similarly, Samuels's breath analyser enabled him to talk about an improvement in his Vo2 max and allow him to present himself as someone who is relatively very fit for his age.

The Production of Fluid Selves

In what ways, then, is Barad's theory of agential realism a useful and provocative way of rethinking notions of how the self is *done* using self-quantifying technologies? As I have argued above, agential realism provides a radical departure from previous theories of the self which deal with performativity and agency. The foundation for Barad's theory is quantum mechanics and a specific set of experiments within that field: the double-slit experiments. This diffractive methodology that she employs, however, is not without faults. Take Barad's example of the nature of the electron as being akin to the self. There is a problem with taking the electron and the 'self' as being comparable. When the electron creates its own photon and then absorbs it, it absorbs it in its entirety. It does not make choices about which part of the photon to absorb, it does not reject certain photons, and it certainly does not try to reconfigure the photon.

The case of the self with respect to self-quantifying technologies is rather different. The self that is created through the self-quantifying technologies is negotiated. Sometimes, the technology is absorbed entirely and enveloped into the self, as was the case with Tamara feeling worse about her ride after she quantified it, and Ben changing his narrative upon seeing the reading on the device. At other times, however, the technology is rejected, moulded, reinterpreted or discarded. There are certain moments where people may 'negotiate' with the technology or the reading on the device. Leo, for example, decided to disregard the advice on his Garmin watch and go for a run anyway. What is apparent, though, is that these technologies are *productive* of the self rather than merely descriptive. They go some way in performing the self by both producing differences that matter and also enabling/constraining what can be said about the self.

What is also apparent here is that the self is not a fixed and stable entity. It appears from my interviews and observations that the self is much more fluid and changeable. Does it make sense, then, to continue to talk about the 'self' as a singular and fixed entity rather than talking of constantly producing and performing 'selves', where the boundaries are increasingly being broadened to allow for things not traditionally included, such as self-quantifying technologies? For example, the self that I was interacting with before Ben's blood glucose device contradicted his intuitions was instantly different to the self after the blood glucose device had given its reading. Similar things can be said about Leo's run after the watch told him that he should rest for 3 days, and his admission that he had felt as though he was totally missing a gear, about Tamara's experience of her commute to work, and about Samuel who physically and mentally felt like a 30-year-old.

Conclusion

Using the case of the Quantified Self, I have shown how the theory of agential realism, with particular reference to the concepts of intra-action and agential cutting, is a useful starting point to thinking about the role of self-quantifying technologies in the way that the 'self' comes to the fore in certain contexts. The concepts of 'discourse' and 'apparatus' allow us to see how self-quantifying technologies can enable/constrain what can be said about the self, as well as how they come to produce differences that matter. And in this context, what matters is the self. In being productive of the self, self-quantifying technologies are implicated in the process of 'agential cutting'—that is, the process of making boundaries around that which comes to be known as the 'self' in that moment. For instance, in enabling Samuel to say that his Vo2 max had increased from 23 ml/kg/min to over 30 ml/kg/min, the Vo2 measuring breath analyser is complicit in the production of a self that has improved. In constraining Ben's ability to talk about a 'light in carbohydrates lunch', his blood glucose monitor is a fundamental part of the production of a self that has high levels of blood glucose and so on.

If, as I have found, these technologies are a fundamental part of the production of fluid and multiple selves with differing narratives of health, illness, positivity or negativity about certain behaviours, then this idea has interesting resonances with discourses on neoliberalism and associated ideas of self-governance. How might these technologies be appropriated by others to achieve wider political ends? For example, might they be used to facilitate shifts towards community-based health care, or austerity cost savings? Might some of the solutions towards self-directed care be more about consumers spending money than citizens improving their health? Whilst these questions were not the focus of this chapter, others have certainly taken on this mode of analysis. Lupton (2014), for example, focuses on what she calls the 'neoliberal political orientation' in which she argues that self-quantification technologies and the algorithms present within them normalise certain kinds of behaviour as the status quo, whilst at the same time putting the responsibility and labour of taking care of oneself onto the individual rather than on the state.

What this chapter has shown, though, is that these self-quantifying technologies seem to be facilitating a new boundary around that which we would traditionally call the 'self'. And this 'self' is not a single, fixed entity, but something that is continually being enacted as it envelops these self-quantifying technologies, which, at the same time, are producing this self. This is where the role of agential cutting becomes important, since this is the mechanism by which this rather fluid and changing concept of the self becomes momentarily stable and has the appearance of being fixed. Rather than self-quantifying technologies reflecting a stable self already out there waiting to be depicted through the data they produce, I proffer the idea that the self-quantifying technologies *are* the multiple enactments of the self and thus cannot be separated from the practices of using them.

References

Austin, J. (1962). *How to do things with words*. Oxford: Clarendon Press.
Barad, K. (2003). Posthumanist Performativity: Toward an understanding of how matter comes to matter. *Signs: Journal of Women in Culture and Society, 28*(3), 801–831.
Barad, K. (2007). *Meeting the universe halfway: Quantum physics and the entanglement of matter and meaning*. Durham & London: Duke University Press.
Barad, K. (2012). Intra-actions. *Mousse, 34,* 76–81.
Barad, K. (2013). On touching-the inhuman that therefore I am. *Differences, 23*(3), 206–223.
Bohr, N. (1935). Can quantum-mechanical description of physical reality be considered complete? *Physical Review, 48,* 696–702.
Butler, J. (1993). *Bodies that matter: On the discursive limits of "Sex"*. London: Routledge.
Butler, J. (2010). Performative agency. *Journal of Cultural Economy, 3*(2), 147–161.
Butler, J. (2013). Acts and gender performative an essay in phenomenology and feminist theory. *Theatre Journal, 40*(4), 519–531.
Einstein, A., Podolsky, B., & Rosen, N. (1935). Can quantum-mechanical description of physical reality be considered complete? *Physical Review, 47,* 777–780.
Festinger, L. (1957). *A theory of cognitive dissonance*. Stanford: Stanford University Press.
Goffman, E. (1959). *The presentation of self in everyday life*. Harmondsworth: Penguin.
Law, J., & Singleton, V. (2000). Performing technology's stories: On social constructivism, performance, and performativity. *Technology and Culture, 14*(4), 765–775.
Lupton, D. (2013). The digitally engaged patient: Self-monitoring and self-care in the digital health era. *Social Theory & Health,* 1–15.
Lupton, D. (2014). Critical perspectives on digital health technologies. *Sociology Compass, 8*(12), 1344–1359.

Mialet, H. (2012). *Hawking incorporated: Stephen Hawking and the anthropology of the knowing subject*. Chicago: University of Chicago Press.

Swan, M. (2009). Emerging patient-driven health care models: An examination of health social networks, consumer personalized medicine and quantified self-tracking. *International Journal of Environmental Research and Public Health, 6*(2), 492–525.

Wolf, G. (2011). 'Quantified Sel' | aether. Available at: http://aether.com/quantifiedself. Accessed November 3, 2011.

Woolgar, S. (2014). Struggles with representation: Could it be otherwise? In C. Coopmans, J. Vertesi, M. Lynch, & S. Woolgar (Eds.), *Representation in scientific practice revisited*. Cambridge: The MIT Press.

Part III
Reconstructing the Medical: Data, Ethics, Discourse and Pmds

The medical aspect of Pmds might be thought to imply a narrowly defined, tightly circumscribed clinical interaction between a user and a device. From this perspective, PMD usage might be expected to occur within accustomed pathways of biomedical institutional hierarchies. However, such a focus overlooks extra-clinical spheres of critical relevance to how Pmds are used in practice and their wider implications for selves, healthcare and society. Chapter 6 considers how the data generated by 'artificial pancreas' systems for people with type 1 diabetes lead to metaphysical and epistemological transformations for users of this PMD, enabling both liberating and constraining aspects of bodily experience. By foregrounding the sensemaking processes of individual PMD users, this chapter reveals how data generated by Pmds outside clinical contexts can reconstitute attitudes to the self and technology. Chapter 7 considers keepsake ultrasounds as a kind of PMD in order to explore the relationship between morality and medicine. In doing so, this chapter reveals how Pmds can unsettle established ethical boundaries and question the moral specialness of medicine while raising new questions for regulatory authorities. Chapter 8, lastly, shifts focus to public debate and discourse surrounding particular Pmds, their predicted use, and estimated impact on health and medicine. This chapter considers e-cigarettes as PMDs in order to highlight how different perspectives within debates about smoking construct e-cigarettes as different objects, such that 'riskiness' can be seen to be a constructed rather than an inherent property. As such, public discourse and debates about PMDs are themselves examples of how new technologies create new relations and material effects that raise important questions about what 'the medical' and the medical is 'done' within wider social contexts.

6

Data as Transformational: Constrained and Liberated Bodies in an 'Artificial Pancreas' Study

Conor Farrington

Introduction

Many personal medical devices (Pmds) generate data about people's movements, activities, and bodily status. Whether intervening within bodies or monitoring them externally, Pmds are a uniquely intimate and ubiquitous source of data, in many cases offering PMD users the ability to gain granular knowledge about hitherto unknown aspects of their own bodies. This chapter foregrounds the specific kinds of data generated about individual patients' bodies by the 'artificial pancreas'. The artificial pancreas system comprises a set of interlinked, body-mounted devices that sense varying interstitial glucose levels in users with type 1 diabetes and utilise machine-learning control algorithms to calculate and administer basal insulin in response to these glucose levels. This system generates precise data regarding insulin dosage and (especially) glucose levels,

C. Farrington (✉)
School of Clinical Medicine, University of Cambridge, Cambridge,
England, UK
e-mail: Cjtf2@medschl.cam.ac.uk

© The Author(s) 2018
R. Lynch and C. Farrington (eds.), *Quantified Lives and Vital Data*,
Health, Technology and Society, https://doi.org/10.1057/978-1-349-95235-9_6

providing significantly greater detail regarding the latter than is available using standard glucose monitoring methods. Through analysis of interviews conducted with participants in a recent overnight study of the 'artificial pancreas' system for pregnant women with type 1 diabetes, this chapter draws on and extends theories of 'sensemaking' (Weick 1995) to explore how PMD data can reconstitute micro-scale attitudes to the self and technology. These transformations can occur at the epistemological level (e.g. through the revelation of unsuspected micro-scale glucose fluctuations) as well as at the metaphysical level, e.g. through the practice-based experience of living as the subject of automated, algorithm-driven treatment. Moreover, these transformations can be both constraining and liberating in different ways, offering new potential for action and improved self-care at the same time as generating new kinds of challenges and problems to be overcome. Consequently, this chapter demonstrates the multiple and complex ways in which data—a somewhat intangible resource, yet also a ubiquitous and personal one—increasingly play important roles in technology-mediated experiences of health and illness. As such, this chapter considers diabetes-related technologies in a different way from Hess (this volume), which focuses on a specific diabetes device—the insulin pump—and considers this device as a visual and material mediator between selves and others. Moreover, while Hess considers devices used in everyday settings, this chapter considers the rather different context represented by pregnant women participating in a medical trial—i.e. a temporary and high-stakes medical condition (pregnancy) in which participants encounter new technology in a highly structured manner and with extensive additional medical and technological support. This context may have affected participant experiences in numerous ways, for instance, by enabling participants to have more positive experiences of new technologies than may have been the case in less supportive environments.

Diabetes and Data

Type 1 diabetes is a chronic condition which requires continuous self-management, usually undertaken by individuals in conjunction with clinical teams in primary or (more often) secondary care settings and often supported with structured education programmes including (in the UK context) DAFNE, or 'dose adjustment for normal eating'. Self-management of diabetes entails a wide range of tasks, which can be grouped (following Hinder and Greenhalgh 2012) into two, often overlapping, categories: *practical-cognitive* tasks (e.g. monitoring glucose levels, assessing nutritional content of food, calculating, and administering insulin) and *socio-emotional* tasks (e.g. coping with feelings about diabetes, making sense of clinical advice, and explaining diabetes to friends and relatives). Many people with diabetes use a range of PMDs to treat their condition, including syringes or pens (both disposable and refillable) for injecting insulin, wearable continuous glucose monitoring (CGM) sensors and receivers (which can measure interstitial glucose levels up to three hundred times a day), and wearable continuous subcutaneous insulin infusion (CSII) pumps (commonly referred to simply as insulin pumps). These PMDs vary significantly in terms of complexity, cost, and capacities, ranging from multiple daily injections (MDI) to the most recent artificial pancreas systems, which combine CGM sensors and CSII pumps with a control algorithm to compute optimal insulin dosage of basal insulin (i.e. insulin delivered overnight and between user-controlled meal boluses during the day; Thabit et al. 2015). Model predictive control (MPC) algorithms for artificial pancreas systems, such as the system discussed here, incorporate a range of complex mathematical models of glucoregulatory systems including insulin-absorption dynamics, insulin-action dynamics, meal-absorption dynamics, plasma-glucose dynamics, and sensor dynamics (Haidar 2016). A number of systems also incorporate machine-learning elements within adaptive algorithms, allowing systems to adapt in real time to high levels of intra- and inter-patient variability in insulin needs and absorption rates (Youssef et al. 2011).

In addition to high levels of variability in terms of physiological response to diabetes, previous research on diabetic technologies attests to significant levels of variability between individuals in terms of the uptake, usage, and effectiveness of CGM sensors and insulin pumps, and suggests that people with diabetes do not always engage sustainably with technological interventions (Raccah et al. 2009). For example, research on CGM sensors in adolescents has highlighted concerns such as painful sensor insertions, increased planning and maintenance requirements, and alarm caused by system notifications and warnings (Rashotte et al. 2014). Anxiety arising from challenges such as these may be heightened by the 'high-stakes' context of pregnancy, in which foetal health is affected as well as maternal health, and by the use of complex and partially automated systems such as artificial pancreas systems (as witnessed by a 10% attrition rate owing to system non-acceptance in a recent major study; Thabit et al. 2015). These challenges may lead to 'diabetes burnout', a condition in which reduced self-management leads to adverse clinical outcomes (Polonsky 1999). Furthermore, research in other fields has demonstrated that technological encounters are generally context-dependent, frequently leading to unpredictable and variable outcomes (Orlikowski and Gash 1994). Consequently, while new diabetic technologies (such as artificial pancreas systems) undoubtedly offer new capacities and new kinds of data, it cannot be assumed that these new capacities will inevitably lead to improved self-care and lowered diabetes-related anxiety. While some researchers have begun to consider these issues with regard to artificial pancreas systems (e.g. Barnard et al. 2014), more research is needed to explore the intricacies of real-life user experience of such systems (Farrington 2015). This is especially the case since, as Hinder and Greenhalgh (2012, p. 2) state, patients with diabetes spend only around 1% of their time in contact with clinical teams; the remaining 99% of patients' time, consequently, is 'virtually a closed book to clinicians and researchers'. As noted above, however, it should be born in mind that the women discussed in this chapter were participants in a medical trial and thus enjoyed higher levels of contact than ordinary patients (though still with very extensive periods of time out of contact with clinicians).

Sensemaking

In order to investigate patients' interactions with data generated by artificial pancreas systems, this chapter draws upon the 'sensemaking' approach developed within organisational sociology by Karl Weick (1995). Weick's approach focuses on how individuals seek to understand—'make sense' of—the world around them by drawing upon their pre-existing identities and 'frames' (a broad concept encompassing individuals' socially shaped knowledge, experience, values, beliefs, assumptions, attitudes, and priorities). Individuals' attempts to reach an understanding of their context occur simultaneously with the generation and alteration, or 'enactment', of these same contexts: '(inter-) actions generate meaning and simultaneously enact the environment that people try to make sense of' (Hultin and Mahring 2016, p. 4). This binding together of sense and action, leading to the construction of (amendable) features of given settings, echoes dominant concerns of structurationist approaches to social ontology (e.g. Giddens 1984). While sensemaking occurs continually, it is particularly to the fore, on Weick's account, when individuals encounter new and unexpected stimuli (such as new technological systems). Each new stimulus typically exhibits varied 'affordances'—i.e. the aspects and features of events, subjects, and objects that allow for different interpretations and actions, defined by Hutchby (2001; cited Bansler and Havn 2006, p. 63) as 'functional and relational aspects which frame, while not determining, the possibilities for agentic action in relation to an object [or situation]'. (This concept is also discussed by Faulkner, this volume.)

While his work is primarily located in organisational research, Weick is attuned to the 'material influence' of technology's affordances as well as the 'meanings associated with them' (1995, pp. 176–177), thus opening space for engagement with other branches of social thought that foreground technology and materiality (e.g. actor-network theory, SCOT, post-humanism, 'thing' studies). Recognising that affordances influence but do not dictate individuals' reactions to specific technologies, Weick insists that agents actively construct technologies rather than passively discovering them. Indeed, for Weick, action is one of the most important differentiators between sensemaking and other, related but distinct, phenomena such as cognition, perception, representation, and interpretation. Nevertheless, Weick has been subject to critiques of excessive cognitivism, on the grounds that he breaks up sense and action and thus subjects and objects. Arguably, this approach perpetuates binary ontological divides that can be read as favouring a voluntarist approach in which human agents are prioritised above material objects and technologies (Hultin and Mahring 2016). Consequently,

Weick's organisational, interactional sensemaking risks collapsing into the alternative, cognitivist approach to sensemaking that has been developed in human–computer interaction research (e.g. Russell et al. 1993; Dervin 1998)—with a concomitant abstract, non-agential, and 'punctualising' approach to technology and materiality (Law 1992; Sandberg and Tsoukas 2015). I return to this critique below. Putting aside the tension between cognitivist and social/interactional aspects in Weick's approach for the moment, it is clear that the voluntarist, agential, and constructionist accents in Weick's theorising point towards a perspectival interpretation of materiality that emphasises multiple potential interpretations of an identical object or technology. This is fleshed out in terms of 'equivocality', which Weick defines as the 'confusion created by two or more meanings' (1995, pp. 176–177), where such meanings—and the actions that may follow from them—appear equally valid. Faced with equivocality, Weick suggests that individuals draw upon their identities and frames in an attempt to impose a less ambiguous interpretation upon equivocal signals and thus provide the basis for action in uncertain circumstances by creating a 'good story' that 'holds disparate elements together long enough to energise and guide action' (1995, pp. 60–61).

More generally, Weick glosses the sensemaking process in terms of agents 'structuring the unknown' by placing new stimuli (e.g. incongruous events, surprising happenings, or crises) into plausible 'maps' through which the world can more easily be understood, acted within, and changed. The act of mapping, which can be read as a cognitivist and even objectivist exercise, is understood by Weick as providing 'hope, confidence, and the means to move from anxiety to action' (Ancona 2011, p. 6; also Weick 2001). Importantly, Weick sees these attempts to reduce ambiguity as proceeding via *plausibility* rather than *accuracy*. In this context, he relates the story of a group of Swiss soldiers who, having got lost in the Alps, successfully navigated home with a map later discovered to be a map of the Pyrenees: 'when you are lost, any old map will do' (1995, p. 54; see below). He also remarks, with regard to technologies and technological objects, that '[b]ecause "objects" have multiple meanings and significance, it is more crucial to get some interpretation to start with than to postpone action until "the" interpretation surfaces' (1995, p. 57). The likelihood of different individuals finding different interpretations plausible (and thus creating different plausible maps) means that equivocality can easily lead to 'multifinality'. In the sensemaking context, multifinality refers to the possibility of multiple and varied outcomes arising from different individuals' experiences of similar situations and contexts. As a tradition of thought, sensemaking thus resonates strongly with sociological research in technological fields, which frequently emphasises themes of constructionism, variability, and unpredictable outcomes of technology usage (Matthewman 2011; Orlikowski and Gash 1994).

Weick's work has been subject to commentaries of various kinds, ranging from elaborations of constructive engagements between critical theory and sensemaking (Mills et al. 2010) to strong critiques questioning Weick's scholarly integrity and rigour (Basboll 2010), as well as the aforementioned concern that sensemaking reproduces binary distinctions and thus risks collapsing into an excessively cognitivist approach. In the light of this latter concern, practice scholars have sought to move Weickian sensemaking away from a dualistic ontology (persons and objects) towards a more post-humanist approach. A practice approach to sensemaking simultaneously builds on and extends beyond recent research which has sought to include non-human actors in analyses of interactive engagement (e.g. Oborn et al. 2013).

Previous sensemaking research can be read as embodying a weak form of relationality. In this approach, while both people and material objects are conceptualised as agents, these two categories are nevertheless conceived as essentially different and separate. This leads to a view in which humans 'as actors ultimately [decide] how they will respond to materiality' and are thus accorded 'the privilege of being the prime authors of meaning and of their own subjectivity… [thus] losing sight of the performative process through which they become conditioned to act and interact in specific ways' (Hultin and Mahring 2016, p. 5). Drawing on Michel Foucault and Judith Butler, Hultin & Mahring propose instead a performative concept of practice as ongoing and relational, foregrounding the 'entangled relationship between "the social" and "the material"', which implies studying practices as always material-discursive' (2016, p. 2). From this point of view, neither the social nor the material is articulated, or articulable, in the absence of the other. As Matthewman (2011, p. 173) states, 'we have always been posthuman'—i.e. we have always and ubiquitously—and thus in large part invisibly—been entangled with our multiple technologies. In this chapter, the performative slant of practice-based sensemaking informs my analysis of how women's experiences of using an artificial pancreas system—and specifically the data produced by the system—undermine essentialist views of the subject as an 'autonomous… and stable entity' (Hultin and Mahring 2016, p. 7). Instead of this static view, this chapter reveals how individuals become enacted and transformed through practices—in this case, through practices of technology use—and experience liberating and constraining dynamics as a result.

Study Context

The study under discussion was a randomised study to assess the feasibility, utility, safety, and efficacy of automated overnight closed-loop (artificial pancreas) insulin delivery at home in women with type 1 diabetes during pregnancy. As with most other kinds of artificial pancreas systems, the study system comprised a wearable CGM sensor with wireless transmitter and hand-held receiver, a platform device (in this case a tablet) mounting an MPC control algorithm with machine-learning elements which calculated optimal insulin dosage in response to CGM readings each night, and a body-mounted, wirelessly controlled insulin pump which titrated and administered subcutaneous insulin.

The principal data generated by the artificial pancreas system used in the study were of two kinds: data on glucose levels and data on insulin dosage. Various read-outs were available to users, including insulin pump read-out of current and past insulin dosage; hand-held CGM receiver with current and recent glucose levels (and predicted rise/fall/ continuity of levels in the near future); and the tablet read-out, which combines these two sources of data into a single read-out.

This chapter focuses instead on the qualitative data generated through semi-structured interviews with 16 pregnant women before and after their participation in the trial, leading to a total of 32 interviews. The interview topic guide sought to account for the potential differences in technology usage arising from patient interactions with this new kind of system, as opposed to more familiar and well-tried devices such as the insulin pumps discussed by Hess (this volume). A thematic analysis approach was utilised to analyse the data (Braun and Clarke 2006), involving six distinct stages: familiarisation with the data; generating initial codes; searching for themes; reviewing themes; defining and naming themes; and producing a final analysis.

Findings: Transformed, Liberated, and Constrained Bodies

This section presents the findings of the study in terms of users' experiences of artificial pancreas technology, with particular regard to how data produced through the use of an automated, algorithm-controlled system can be understood as facilitating a number of different processes, experiences, and sensemaking approaches. The findings presented here focus in particular upon two key aspects of data in the context of the artificial pancreas study which formed the backdrop of this research agenda. The first section, 'Transformed Bodies', focuses on the ways in which use of artificial pancreas systems led to shifts in users' epistemological and metaphysical conceptions of their diabetic bodies. Far from viewing the subject as stable, fixed, or autonomous, this section reveals how technology-stimulated sensemaking led to new kinds of subjective experience and practices. The second section, 'Constrained and Liberated Bodies', shifts the focus to the implications of these transformations and practices in different dimensions and for different women. While artificial pancreas technology in some ways enabled liberating experiences for some women and at some times, for other women, and in other ways and times, it led to experiences that were more constraining than enabling. In line with a practice-based sensemaking approach, that is, these findings suggest that technologies, like subjects, cannot be considered in terms of unchanging, inherent, and essential properties that exert uniform effects.

Transformed Bodies

Epistemological transformations, which are considered first, tended to be associated with data on glucose levels generated by wearable CGM sensors, whereas metaphysical transformations tended to be associated with data relating to insulin dosage and, more widely, users' reactions to being controlled by a machine—or, more specifically, the control algorithm located on the study tablet in conjunction with a body-mounted insulin pump.

Epistemological Transformations

In terms of epistemological transformations, first, it is worth noting the backdrop against which many participants discussed their changed attitudes arising from data. Diabetes, as noted above, is a chronic disorder requiring the constant enactment of self-management in terms of diet, exercise, and insulin dosage, and with significant additional burdens arising during pregnancy as a result of physiological and lifestyle changes. In this context, interviewees frequently emphasised the need for people with diabetes to live 'quantified lives', encompassing a range of burdensome, time-consuming activities centred upon the classification of key dimensions of self-care in numerical terms. One interviewee discussed this issue with particular reference to exercise:

> It's time-consuming… the impact of diabetes on my life means things like, if my friends go, do you want to go for a run? I'll go, oh okay, hang on, let me just check how my blood sugars are; how long are we going to be running for? How fast are we going to be running? And then I just take all these things into consideration, put that into my pump, work out roughly, do, like, mental arithmetic on how much to reduce my insulin by to allow my blood sugars to rise enough. So it's constantly numbers going round in your head.

More widely, interviewees alluded to the quotidian processes of quantification associated with diabetes, including blood glucose self-testing (using finger-prick strips), 'carb-counting' (establishing the carbohy-drate content in food), and the estimated impact of particular activities (e.g. work, exercise, sleep) on future glucose levels. For some interview-ees, these activities were mentioned in a positive light, with regard to the knowledge that they generated about the body and its response to external factors such as exercise and insulin therapy; thus, one woman stated: 'Yeah, I like to understand, obviously it's my body, it's happening to me, it's going on inside me, so therefore I like to know'.

For most participants, however, these necessary tasks were more often discussed in terms of the burdens they involve and specifically with regard to the challenges they pose in terms of living a 'normal' life (i.e. a life without diabetes). In this context, one participant described the various self-management activities associated with diabetes as having a 'massive' impact on her daily life:

> You have to think about everything you eat, all the activity you do, how it's going to affect your blood sugars, just the smallest tasks can make a big difference depending what your blood glucose is. So it has a massive impact.

A related concern, which several women raised with regard to checking glucose levels, was the way in which diabetic self-care activities could simultaneously remind the sufferer of their disorder and advertise its presence to others. Thus, one interviewee stated that 'the worst thing about it is it reminds you that you're diabetic [and] you're telling every-body else. It's almost like… why does anybody else need to know'.

The technological and clinical advances represented by artificial pancreas systems—and the quotidian sensemaking practices involved in their use—need to be considered against this backdrop of continu-ous self-care activities related to quantification. In particular, the near-continuous glucose data afforded by CGM sensor systems represent a very considerable augmentation of data in terms of quantity, offering almost 300 readings per day as opposed to the 4–8 finger-prick readings a person with diabetes might undertake with conventional MDI insu-lin therapy. In one sense, this augmentation relates to a shift in degree rather than in kind, since glucose is still measured invasively—albeit in this case through a continuously inserted subcutaneous sensor rather than the momentary piercing of the skin with a hand-held lancet required for finger-prick testing—and still produces a number of readings per day. In another sense, however, the CGM readings generated by the artificial pancreas system are so frequent as to represent a different kind of knowledge about the body than is possible with finger-prick testing alone, and additionally a kind of knowledge generated with somewhat less negative impact on daily life than finger-prick testing (though some finger-prick blood tests are required to calibrate each new sensor).

The additional data presented by CGM readings could be confusing or bewildering at first. For example, one interviewee stated that the CGM data were 'amazing, yeah, a bit of a head spinner, because it was testing my blood every five minutes and I wasn't quite used to seeing patterns like that so often'. For most interviewees, however, these highly detailed and granular data led to transformations in how they viewed their own bodies. The artificial pancreas system generated additional data points that illuminated their bodies' responses to food, activity, and insulin, and which also constituted substantive guides to future action (as discussed in the following section). One interviewee described the knowledge she gained from the CGM data with regard to her response to physical exercise in particular:

> I always thought that I reacted, you know, I was quite sensitive to exercise, but actually when we had the sensor, we realised that it didn't have that much of an impact, but I did have lows a lot later, so within the 24 hours I could go lower. So I didn't really realise that before, because I hadn't had, sort of, the data to see it.

Relatedly, a number of study participants emphasised the insights that CGM data offered in terms of their body's reactions to food and other external factors. One interviewee, for example, described how she was surprised by CGM data on her reaction to specific foods: 'if I ate lots of pasta, for instance, I remember, then my sugars would stay high for quite a long time, a lot longer after the meal than I would have thought'. These data also provided surprises in terms of temporary peaks and troughs in glucose that seemingly occurred for no obvious reason, as one woman described: 'last night, I didn't have any reason for it to go up to 12 but it went up to 12 for no reason... It's surprising how sitting around makes your sugars go up'.

Overall, the CGM data generated by patients' use of the artificial pancreas system in their enactments of self-care led to significant epistemological shifts in how participants regarded their bodies, leading to large advances in participants' ability to understand their bodies' reactions to food, exercise, and other behavioural factors. Additionally, CGM data offered reassurance and confirmation of women's own perceptions of their glucose levels and allowed for much easier access to data than available through conventional (finger-prick) methods. One interviewee summed up her transformational view of the CGM data as follows:

> The CGM was amazing. It was like, it's like being completely blind and then having somebody open your eyes... It puts the power back into your hands because it's all going on inside of you.

Metaphysical Transformations

While the preceding section focused on epistemological transformations arising from glucose data generated by CGM sensors, this section focuses on metaphysical transformations arising from CGM data in addition to data on automatically administered insulin dosage. These transformations are here understood in terms of participants' perceptions of themselves as part human, part machine hybrids (or 'cyborgs'; Haraway 1985)—perceptions that arose because of the sense in which elements of the artificial pancreas system are both subcutaneously inserted into and effectively 'control' key aspects of participants' bodies.

In this context, several interviewees discussed feelings of reluctance that frequently arose when they first utilised wearable, subcutaneously inserted diabetic technologies such as insulin pumps, CGM sensors, or both (in the context of artificial pancreas systems). These feelings related to both concerns about human–machine hybridity itself (e.g. a disinclination to be 'hooked up' to a machine) and concerns about the reliability and safety of intensive insulin therapy delivered by an algorithm-controlled system. In terms of the former, several interviewees mentioned a reluctance to have a device attached to their bodies at all times, stating (for instance) that 'I didn't like the idea of having something attached to me the whole time and I just didn't like the idea of it... I just thought it would make you feel a bit like a robot'. For some participants, this reluctance arose in part because of their sense that wearable diabetic technologies would serve as a constant reminder of the condition, stating (for example) that 'I hate the idea of being attached to something 24/7 'cause it's a reminder that I've got diabetes'. For others, more pragmatic concerns dominated, relating, for instance, to the problems presented by fitting wearable technology around clothes in warmer weather:

> Now that we're coming into slightly warmer weather, I am finding it really difficult. I like to wear things like dresses, and skirts and tops. And it just feels like its protruding out... I do find it quite restrictive in what I can wear.

However, enactment of diabetic self-care through the use of the artificial pancreas system usually overcame these objections, leading in many cases to an emotional sense of identification with the artificial pancreas system and a sense of wonderment at its clinical capabilities. In terms of identification, several interviewees discussed the process of learning a new technology and the emotion and trust that is frequently invested in new systems by participants. One participant discussed her reluctance to give control of her diabetes to a system until she has personally experienced its effectiveness—a reluctance that derived in large part from her long habits of self-management:

> I felt like I was giving the control to a device and I found that strange because I think, well, for me, you feel like your diabetes, sort of you're in control, do you know what I mean? ... so you're handing that control over to a device that initially you don't have any confidence in.

Another interviewee described this process as potentially fraught with difficulty in the event of technical failure:

> Yeah, I've experienced pump failure… And it's quite scary at the time, because it's this thing that's become, you know, part of your life and you're really dependent on and you trust it and this is all trust and it lets you down and it's, like, no, you cannot let me down, I've let you into my life and I trusted you and look what you've done.

Once the initial reluctance to trust new systems has been overcome, a number of participants reported developing more positive attitudes towards the artificial pancreas system. One interviewee referred to actions carried out by the system as if it were a conscious agent rather than an automated system, for example, with regard to an alarm going off overnight:

> [The] first time it happened during the night it was quite unsettling, because I've had a couple of times in the evenings where I've had [the system] going and, obviously, there's been some sort of issue … and Florence [the study name for the artificial pancreas system] has freaked out and switched back to open loop.

Reflecting Weick's emphasis on technology's 'equivocality' (i.e. its openness to different interpretations), other participants often spoke of the system becoming part of their bodies, with particular reference to the impressive clinical capacities of the devices (the sense of wonderment mentioned above)—a theme that resonates with the practice-based sensemaking focus on social–material entanglements. These capacities were made clear to participants in terms of not just their CGM readings, which indicated the extent to which their glucose levels remained within safe levels, but also the insulin dosage calculated by the control algorithm device in response to the CGM readings. The blue-coloured reading on the study tablet shows participants the real-time responses of the system to their CGM readings, graphically illustrating the extreme responsiveness of the device when compared with a set of 'guesstimated' daily insulin injections. One interviewee described the revelatory character of this read-out (which can also be observed, less clearly, on the insulin pump display) in terms of the 'skyscrapers' drawn by the blue display, indicating the variable levels of insulin administered over time by the system:

> When you look at the graph and... when you see it reacting to the [CGM] trends and it builds these, sort of, sky scrapers and it makes absolute sense and it's phenomenal for your control.

On the basis of these clinical capacities, one interviewee stated how she had come to regard the study devices as a part of her:

> [The system] used to be this thing that used to have to hang on my hip or my trousers or be in my pocket, it used to be a problem to me, it really did, it was a hindrance to start with. ... And I think it just took a couple of weeks, just seeing the difference it made ... And as the blood sugars got better and I felt better I was just like, this is just a part of me.

Yet more fundamentally, several participants described the system as taking the place of a functioning pancreas. Thus, one woman remarked: 'I feel quite safe... I don't know, it's like having a pancreas that works... not waking up [with] high [glucose] is lovely; not waking up needing like a pint of water is lovely'. Another participant stated that using the system had led her to feel as if she were a 'normal person' and not diabetic: 'now, because my blood sugar control is so good and I feel so positive about it it's almost like I'm a normal person and I'm not diabetic'.

Consequently, the data provided by the artificial pancreas system can be seen to occasion metaphysical as well as epistemological transformations, leading participants to overcome their reluctance in terms of wearable devices and bringing them to conceive of the study devices as part of their bodies, as personalised technologies, and as 'replacing' their malfunctioning pancreases, therefore enabling them to live more normal lives. Data generated by the artificial pancreas do not only change the way that users come to know about their bodies, but also change the kinds of things that they think their bodies are. In opposition to a cognitivist interpretation of sensemaking, these findings illustrate the profound entanglement of subject and object, human and technology, patient and artificial pancreas system that participants experienced and enacted in the course of the trial. Far from reproducing 'natural' or static distinctions between the two sides of these and other binaries, these findings illustrate how sensemaking practices, enacted in the course of diabetic self-care, both rest upon and further extend the inextricable and manifold connections between seemingly distinct actors, objects, and contexts.

'Real Bonuses' and 'Little Doubts': Liberated and Constrained Bodies

While the previous section considered the epistemological and metaphysical transformations occasioned by new kinds of data, this section foregrounds the consequences and implications of these transformations for everyday life lived with type 1 diabetes. These implications are considered in terms of liberating and constraining dimensions, understood in terms of factors that expand or restrain human agency, respectively.

Liberated Bodies

Interviewees discussed two principal kinds of improvement arising from the data generated by artificial pancreas systems, focusing on improved self-care possibilities and wider notions of improved lives, respectively. In terms of improved self-care, participants highlighted a number of ways in which CGM and insulin dosage data created new possibilities for managing diabetes on a day-to-day basis. For example, several interviewees emphasised how the CGM data (and related alarms activated on the hand-held CGM receiver device) could supplement and at times supplant the body's own warning signals with regard to impending hypo- or hyperglycaemia. This notion was often phrased in terms of perceptions of impending hypoglycaemia, with real-time data offering the potential to reassure users that their own perceptions were correct. Thus, one interviewee stated that:

It's nice to know what's happening, and also, like matching sometimes, the symptoms, with what's going on in my blood sugar, whereas before I'd have to check my blood sugar every 12 hours, you can actually just look and go, oh I'm not feeling quite right, oh that's why, it's 'cause my blood sugars are starting to go, or, starting to go down.

This reassurance, moreover, was easily available: rather than having to undergo a finger-prick test, study participants were able to check their glucose levels instantly by glancing at the hand-held receiver or tablet study device. A number of interviewees highlighted the value of being able to access glucose levels in this manner, with one woman describing herself as becoming 'obsessed' with looking at the hand-held receiver device:

I've been a bit obsessed looking at that actually because I was always an avid blood sugar tester anyway, so I'd test eight to ten times a day. So the fact that I haven't had to prick my finger that much and I can literally just pick it up and look at it, so particularly at work if I've been busy I've been managing to just have a look at it.

This aspect of the findings reveals, in strikingly tangible terms, the entanglement of subjectivity and materiality (cf Hultin and Mahring 2016) occasioned by user interactions with the artificial pancreas. The ready visibility of glucose levels on the hand-held device led not so much to a new kind of attitude (as this user was already an 'avid tester') so much as a new kind of daily practice, in which finger-pricking has been replaced by looking obsessively at a small screen read-out. (The potential downside of such obsessiveness is considered below.)

The reassurance that users derived from using the system was often linked to notions of *safety*, with particular emphasis laid upon system alarms to alert users of impending or current hypoglycaemia. One interviewee noted how she had struggled to maintain good glucose control in previous pregnancies, a fact which made the artificial pancreas system more attractive:

In my past pregnancies, I've suffered with hypos during the night quite a lot and it was always a constant battle with both of them. So, the opportunity to have a constant glucose monitor to catch when my bloods were going low before they got too low was… a real bonus, to hopefully avoid similar problems that we had in the past.

In addition to improved safety, many participants emphasised the improved control of glucose that arose through the usage of the system. Interestingly, this improved control was not only mentioned with regard to the 'closed-loop' part of the study, in which participants' insulin dosage was controlled overnight by the control algorithm device, but also in terms of the 'open-loop' part of the study, in which participants were responsible for controlling their own insulin dosage via their insulin pumps. In this regard, the CGM data were regarded as crucial for informing more granular and precise self-management routines. Thus, one interviewee stated that 'I think the sensor's brilliant… Because [it] gives you all the information you need to get it right'. Similarly, another woman stated that 'I know what I'm doing, I know where my blood sugar is going so I can act accordingly… it helps you prepare and act accordingly'.

This improved control of glucose was linked by several participants with wider notions of reduced fear and heightened power over their own bodies and care routines. In comments indicating an empowering intertwinement of technology and subjectivity, users felt more in control not just of their glucose levels but of diabetes more widely. As mentioned previously, several participants described how the artificial pancreas system helped them to feel more 'normal' and akin to a person without diabetes. Several participants acknowledged that this was more of an ideal than an attainable reality, but nevertheless expressed the view that new technologies such as the artificial pancreas represent important way stations in this direction—as shown by this participant's statement:

> [E]ven with technology, [diabetes is] always going to hold you back somewhat, but it's just, I think … the technology … limits how much it's going to hold you back by… and with all the new technologies that are coming out, it's getting easier and easier.

In the context of new technologies, a number of interviewees found the experience of participating in the study a stimulating one and derived considerable satisfaction from their successful use of the system to control their diabetes more effectively. For instance, one interviewee stated that 'the only word I can think of [is] it's quite exciting to know that I can learn something like that and make it work'. Other participants expressed the view that new technologies such as the artificial pancreas gave them a more central role in their own care, helping to support a partnership between the patient and doctor rather than a top-down, doctor-first model:

> Even though I have this … disease that's not going to go away, you… feel really, well (a) you're in control, because I'm a control freak, I like to be in control of my own health and (b) it's more a partnership, I don't have to sit cap in hand in a waiting room waiting for, you know, two hours for someone to then give me five minutes of time.

From this perspective, new technologies can be understood not just as specific devices with which particular individuals interact, but as potentially transformative interventions in wider socio-technical networks of care (as previously highlighted in research on telecare; Oudshoorn 2011).

More widely, the same interviewee summed up many of the themes canvassed here with regard to empowerment by suggesting that diabetes technology (like the artificial pancreas system) can transform diabetics' lives for the better: 'it's giving me the information I really need and… I mean, it just transforms your life. I mean, the difference between my life with and without a pump is scarily phenomenal'.

Constrained Bodies

While there is no doubt that the new kinds of data generated by the artificial pancreas system offered participants a range of empowering experiences, they also raised a number of new challenges, which some participants experienced as oppressive, constraining burdens. A number of these challenges arose in domains other than CGM or insulin data, as seen, for instance, in cases where participants had been given differing advice from different clinics regarding the treatment of hypoglycaemia, and in one case in which the participant dropped out of the study because of her dislike of the study insulin pump (which is less user-friendly than some pumps). Some participants also expressed concerns, mentioned above, about being hooked up to and controlled by a machine, while others highlighted the significant burdens that study participation involved, including the logistical challenges of maintaining a complex set of interrelated devices at the same time as managing the challenges of pregnancy, career and family responsibilities, and ongoing requirements relating to diabetic self-care. In this context, participants frequently described the artificial pancreas system as bulky and cumbersome, and frequently alluded to logistical challenges relating to mastering training materials, keeping devices charged, and maintaining connectivity between the devices (which can be difficult in some buildings). In this light, one interviewee described the system as 'quite cumbersome, quite big, lots of wires… it's not really something you could put in your handbag and nip to the shops with'. This kind of challenge echoes the structurationist element of sensemaking, with enacted technological practices enabling new actions and constraining others (Weick 1995).

Participants also raised specific concerns in terms of data, which are the focus of the remainder of this section. These concerns fell into three main categories, relating to concerns of addiction, outsourcing, and unreliability. With regard to addiction, a number of participants expressed general concerns about addiction to technologies and mobile technologies in particular—a concern raised above with regard to the 'obsessive' checking of glucose levels. One participant described technology addiction as limiting the possibilities for mother–child interaction: 'I don't like the whole addiction… I was reading about the young mums where they're not getting their actual physical face time with their children… because they're texting while they're breastfeeding'. A small number of participants also expressed these general concerns more specifically with regard to the hand-held CGM receiver device, while at the same time acknowledging the value of the data:

I think the biggest thing is just being able to see your blood sugars in front of you all of the time, and seeing what they're doing. And, it's actually quite scary to begin with… [but] now, I think, if I were to not have the CGM, as my husband says, you'd miss it, you wouldn't know what to look at. [Interviewer: It becomes almost addictive.] It does, it's a bit like a smart phone, you know.

The same interviewee elaborated further on this theme, suggesting that the compelling nature of the data is linked to its unpredictability and to the anxiety that arises from being able to observe one's own glucose levels in real time:

> I've had the odd time when they've been a little bit unpredictable, and you sit and watch them, and I then start thinking, is it what I've eaten, is it the set, is the set working properly. And, you watch them go up and up and up...

From this perspective, the constant availability of CGM data, and its entwining within everyday sensemaking practices of self-care, can cause anxiety as well as offering reassurance and new ways of knowing about the body.

A different concern arose with regard to 'outsourcing', which is here used to refer to the deskilling process that can occur when users of CGM technology come to rely on the devices to such an extent that they become less aware of bodily sensations that indicate hypo- or hyperglycaemia, such as thirst, fatigue, shakiness, and anxiety. One participant described this process as follows:

> I feel as though my hypo-awareness has dropped, because I think I've become too dependent on the navigator telling me ... I feel as though, rather than being conscious of how I'm feeling all the time, I'll just wait for the navigator to beep and tell me that I'm going to go low.

In this context, another interviewee reported that the artificial pancreas system had made her 'slightly more passive... it definitely made me lazier and slightly more passive in my own care, which is, I guess, not a good thing'. These findings reveal how technology can not only become entangled with the everyday practices of individual users but also transform their sense of their own bodies, in this case simultaneously empowering and constraining individuals by reducing the need for users to pay attention to their feelings and causing a loss of bodily perceptiveness thereby. At the same time, however, other interviewees noted how the CGM sensor could also detect peaks and troughs that were too small-scale or short-lived for them to become aware of themselves. Consequently, the outsourcing, or deskilling, that can occur with new diabetic technologies needs to be weighed against the more granular data that such technologies offer.

Finally, concerns arose about the accuracy of the CGM data and the implications of inaccuracies and sensor failures for levels of trust in the wider artificial pancreas system. A number of interviewees mentioned the variable accuracy of the CGM data and expressed concerns regarding the potentially inaccurate insulin dosage that the artificial pancreas may administer on that basis. One participant stated:

> My only worry – well, my main worry – was with the CGM… because it's not 100 per cent [accurate]… [W]hat if… the pump thinks that my blood sugars are actually this level, but actually they are lower than that… so it either gives me less insulin or it gives me more insulin, and I'm not getting that tight control that I'm thinking I'm going to get by doing this study?

Another participant described her experience of a faulty batch of CGM sensors: 'when it was giving readings it was giving me incorrect readings, and it was telling me that I was going hypo and I really wasn't, and then that made me question, well, am I losing my alertness of hypos coming'. On the basis of these inaccurate readings, she described her overall level of trust in the system as follows: 'I wouldn't say I trust it massively, [around] 50 or 60 per cent… there's always that little doubt in my head… there's always glitches that can happen'.

Challenges such as these, which relate to the process of generating the data and possible implications for the quality of the data generated, had the potential to cause significant disruption and anxiety in participants' lives. One interviewee, for instance, described how her CGM reading had been falsely low overnight, preventing her from sleeping:

> [My] blood sugar last night, was three all night, and it really made me panic. And I couldn't sleep and I just had to keep eating and eating and eating. And it got to four o'clock and I know I should have done it earlier, but I did a finger prick test, and my blood sugar was actually six… I've found that really hard.

Consequently, it is clear that the new kinds of data generated by the artificial pancreas system create new challenges and obstacles as well as new potential for action and self-treatment. As Weick remarks (1995, p. 31): 'people act and in so doing create the materials that become the constraints and opportunities they face'.

Discussion

The findings presented in this chapter show that interviewees experienced a range of transformations as a result of the various kinds of data generated by their use of the artificial pancreas system. For example, users experienced epistemological transformations with regard to their knowledge of their own bodies. The wealth of real-time data on glucose levels generated by CGM sensors not only offered additional insight into their reactions to food and exercise, but was also experienced as an 'eye-opening' shift in self-perception. Metaphysically, study participants were initially reluctant to countenance their transformation into body/machine hybrids owing to practical concerns and anxiety about being controlled by an algorithm at a time when another and even more significant set of bodily transformations—i.e. changes related to pregnancy—were taking place. Most participants, however, came to accept and even embrace this hybridity, with some interviewees mentioning their sense of becoming more 'normal' as a result. Transformations also occurred with regard to empowerment, articulated through notions of reassurance, accessibility, safety, control, and more power over their condition, and with regard to new challenges and problems such as anxiety arising from 'addiction' to CGM data, deskilling of bodily perception through 'outsourcing', and inaccurate data leading to lower levels of trust in the artificial pancreas system.

However, these transformations were not linear or uniform and were not shared in a homogeneous manner across study participants. Interviewees who emphasised epistemological transformations frequently passed over metaphysical transformations with little comment and vice versa. Moreover, while ideas of liberation predominated overall, they were often expressed alongside perceptions of constraint, suggesting that liberation and constraint may best be considered as two sides of the same coin. Related to this, the minority of participants who emphasised oppression were also willing to acknowledge ways in which the artificial pancreas system offered new and empowering possibilities. Consequently, these findings resonate with previous research in sociology which emphasises the complexity and unpredictability of user encounters with technology (Orlikowksi and Gash 1994; Matthewman 2011), and with research in diabetes which recounts variable and often unsustainable experiences of diabetic technologies (Raccah et al. 2009; Rashotte et al. 2014).

These findings also illuminate the value of Weick's sensemaking framework at the same time as emphasising the benefits of more recent practice-based interpretations of this framework. Weick's account of sensemaking, it will be recalled, emphasises how individuals engage in sensemaking when stimulated by uncertainty, such as the equivocality arising from the affordances offered by a new piece of technology (such as the artificial pancreas system). In making sense of new technologies, individuals draw on their identities and 'frames' in order actively to construct plausible maps with which to navigate new actions and experiences (Weick 1995). The need for such maps is especially pressing with complex technological systems such as the artificial pancreas, since they comprise a number of different devices, each of which has already been shown to engender complex and varied user experiences, and each of which offers a range of affordances and capacities. Yet, the pressing need for sensemaking does not entail that each individual will make sense of new technologies in the same way, as demonstrated by the 'multifinality' (multiple outcomes or temporary endpoints) experienced by users in terms of epistemological, metaphysical, liberating, and constraining dimensions of artificial pancreas technologies. Moreover, the sensemaking approach suggests that while different individuals may come to different conclusions in terms of their interpretations of a given piece of technology, it is not necessarily justifiable to critique these interpretations or attempt to adjudicate between them. As Battles et al. (2006, p. 3) state, 'to "make sense" is not to find the "right" or "correct" answer, but to find a pattern, albeit temporary, that gives meaning to the individual or group doing the reflection'. Rather than seeking to utilise data on user experience as the basis for prioritising 'correct' interpretations, the sensemaking approach encourages rather the need for productive engagements with the realities of patient experience of PMD usage in home ('real life') settings.

Yet, these same realities, as revealed in the findings presented above, also point to the limitations of approaches that confine themselves (as Weick's approach arguably does) to 'cognitivist' divides between subject and objects or persons and technologies. Use of artificial pancreas systems led to new kinds of subjective experience and new kinds of practices that, taken together, necessitated a form of analysis that goes beyond a voluntarist focus on humans as 'experiencers' of independent, pre-defined technological objects. Rather, ongoing processes of everyday technological engagement led to new kinds of practice and subjectivity in which users experienced enhanced self-knowledge and anxiety about being a 'robot', feelings of safety, and obsessive checking of glucose levels. By incorporating the artificial pancreas system into their daily self-care practices, users created new kinds of human–technology assemblages with complex implications for enactments of the self. While Weick rightly emphasises the equivocality of technology, practice-based sensemaking approaches also emphasise the equivocality of the subject. Such approaches, that is, acknowledge that neither subjects nor technologies come 'pre-packaged' with essential, inherent, autonomous, and stable properties, but rather emerge through 'the entangled relationship between "the social" and "the material"' (Hultin and Mahring 2016, p. 2). Consequently, by drawing upon the multiple insights generated by sensemaking approaches, this chapter has demonstrated the multiple and complex ways in which data—a somewhat intangible resource, yet also a ubiquitous and personal one—play important and transformational, yet complex and nonlinear, roles in technology-mediated experiences of health and illness.

Acknowledgements I am grateful to Rebecca Lynch for her insightful comments on earlier drafts of this chapter.

Note

All interview material used in this chapter was gained with informed consent and is used with permission.

References

Ancona, D. (2011). Sense-making: Framing and acting in the unknown. In S. Snook et al (eds.), *The Handbook for Teaching Leadership* (pp. 3–20). London: Sage.

Bansler, J. P., & Havn, E. (2006). Sensemaking in technology-use mediation: Adapting groupware technology in organizations. *Computer Supported Cooperative Work, 15,* 55–91.

Battles, J., Dixon, N., Borotkanics, R., et al. (2006). Sensemaking of Patient Safety: Risks and Hazards. *Health Services Research, 41*(4), 1555–1575.

Barnard, K., Wysocki, T., Allen, J., et al. (2014). Closing the loop overnight at home setting: Psychosocial impact for adolescents with type 1 diabetes and their parents. *BMJ Open Diabetes Research & Care.* doi:10.1136/bmjdrc-2014-000025.

Basbøll, T. (2010). Softly constrained imagination: Plagiarism and misprision in the theory of organizational sensemaking. *Culture and Organization, 16*(2), 163–178.

Braun, V., & Clarke, V. (2006). Using thematic analysis in psychology. *Qualitative Research in Psychology, 3*(2), 77–101.

Dervin, B. (1998). Sense-making theory and practice: An overview of user interests in knowledge seeking and use. *Journal of Knowledge Management, 2*(2), 36–46.

Farrington, C. (2015). The artificial pancreas: Challenges and opportunities. *Lancet Diabetes and Endocrinology, 3*(2), 937.

Giddens, A. (1984). *The constitution of society: Outline of the theory of structuration.* Los Angeles: University of California Press.

Haidar, A. (2016). The Artificial Pancreas: How Closed-Loop Control is Revolutionizing Diabetes. *IEEE Control Systems Magazine.* doi:10.1109/MCS.2016.2584318.

Haraway, D. (1985). A manifesto for cyborgs: Science, technology, and socialist feminism in the 1980s. *Socialist Review, 80,* 65–107.

Hinder, S., & Greenhalgh, T. (2012). "This does my head in". Ethnographic study of self-management by people with diabetes. *BMC Health Services Research, 12,* 83. doi:10.1186/1472-6963-12-83.

Hultin, L., & Mahring, M. (2016). How practice *makes* sense in healthcare operations: Studying sensemaking as performative, material-discursive practice. *Human Relations.* doi:10.1177/0018726716661618.

Law, J. (1992). Notes on the theory of the actor-network: Ordering, strategy, and heterogeneity. *Systems Practice, 5*(4), 379–393.

Matthewman, S. (2011). *Technoloy and social theory*. London: Palgrave Macmillan.

Mills, J., Thurlow, A., & Mills, A. (2010). Making sense of sensemaking: The critical sensemaking approach. *Qualitative Research in Organizations and Management, 5*(2), 182–195.

Oborn, E., Barrett, M., & Dawson, S. (2013). Distributed leadership in policy formulation: A sociomaterial perspective. *Organization Studies, 34*(2), 253–276.

Orlikowski, W., & Gash, D. (1994). Technological frames: Making sense of information technology in organizations. *ACM Transactions of Information Systems, 12*(2), 174–207.

Oudshoorn, N. (2011). *Telecare technologies and the transformation of healthcare*. London: Palgrave Macmillan.

Polonsky, W. (1999). *Diabetes burnout*. Alexandria, VA: American Diabetes Association.

Raccah, D., Sulmont, V., Reznik, Y., et al. (2009). Incremental value of continuous glucose monitoring when starting pump therapy in patients with poorly controlled type 1 diabetes. *Diabetes Care, 32,* 2245–2250.

Rashotte, J., Tousignant, K., Richardson, C., et al. (2014). Living with sensor-augmented pump therapy in type 1 diabetes: Adolescents' and parents' search for harmony. *Canadian Journal of Diabetes, 38*(4), 256–262.

Russell, M., Stefik, M., Pirolli, P., & Card S. (1993). The cost structure of sensemaking. In *CHI Proceedings of the INTERACT 93 and CHI 93 Conference on Human Factors in Computing Systems* (pp. 269–276). Amsterdam: ACM.

Sandberg, J., & Tsoukas, H. (2015). Making sense of the sensemaking perspective: Its constituents, limitations, and opportunities for further development. *Journal of Organizational Behavior, 36*(S1), S6–S32.

Thabit, H., Tauschmann, M., Allen, J., et al. (2015). Home use of an artificial beta cell in type 1 diabetes. *New England Journal of Medicine*. doi:10.1056/NEJMoa1509351.

Weick, K. (1995). *Sensemaking in organizations*. Thousand Oaks, CA: Sage.

Weick, K. (2001). *Making Sense of the Organization*. Oxford: Blackwell.

Youssef, E. l., Castle, J. R., Branigan, D. L., Massoud, R. G., Breen, M. E., Jacobs, P. G., et al. (2011). "A controlled study of the effectiveness of an adaptive closed-loop algorithm to minimize corticosteroid-induced stress hyperglycemia in type 1 diabetes." *Journal of Diabetes Science and Technology*, Vol. 5, (pp. 1312–1326).

7

PMDs and the Moral Specialness of Medicine: An Analysis of the 'Keepsake Ultrasound'

Anna Smajdor and Andrea Stöckl

Introduction: Keepsake Ultrasound as PMD

In this chapter, we examine the threats that PMDs pose to medicine through their capacity to highlight inconsistencies between attitudes to risk and responsibility when framed as 'medical' or 'non-medical'. The application of special protocols to items demarcated as 'medical' is based on a fundamental precept of medical ethics: first, do no harm. It is also rooted in the idea that medicine is essentially *different* from other endeavours. The proliferation of devices that cross the boundary between medical and non-medical raises ethical questions about the moral

A. Smajdor (✉)
Department of Philosophy, Classics, History of Art and Ideas,
University of Oslo, Oslo, Norway
e-mail: anna.smajdor@ifikk.uio.no

A. Stöckl
Norwich Medical School, University of East Anglia,
Norwich, UK
e-mail: a.stockl@uea.ac.uk

© The Author(s) 2018
R. Lynch and C. Farrington (eds.), *Quantified Lives and Vital Data*,
Health, Technology and Society, https://doi.org/10.1057/978-1-349-95235-9_7

specialness of medicine. It also poses a challenging dichotomy of values. Should we respect people's choices concerning their use of PMDs? Or should we intervene to protect people from the harm that may be caused by 'medical' devices when used for 'non-medical' purposes?

We focus on the case of foetal ultrasound undertaken for non-medical purposes: so-called keepsake ultrasound (Leung and Pang 2009). There is currently little data on how many women use keepsake ultrasound or why. However, sociologist Roberts and colleagues published useful research in 2015. Forty-eight women were recruited from two British commercial ultrasound companies over a period of 11 months (Roberts et al. 2015). The women recruited gave various reasons for their interest in keepsake ultrasound. Many stated that the routine ultrasounds provided on the NHS were very quick. The keepsake ultrasound gave them an opportunity to spend longer over the process and to control the timing. The need for reassurance was also mentioned as being important. The researchers quote one participant who suggested that all pregnant women would have an ultrasound every day if they could. Participants also emphasised the importance of scans as a part of good parenting, especially in terms of allowing parents to connect with their baby before its birth.

An ultrasound image is not obviously a device per se, but for the purposes of our discussion, we construe the keepsake ultrasound as a PMD. This is because an ultrasound image, like an X-ray, can be regarded as an artefact that is the product of a medical procedure, which in turn can be medically interpreted to yield a diagnosis. In the case of medically provided ultrasound, the image has an additional function which is often alluded to by healthcare professionals in patient information literature: by enabling parents to see the baby, it may facilitate bonding (U.S. Food and Drug Administration 2015). As suggested by Roberts et al., it is often this latter function that attracts people who access keepsake ultrasound outside the clinic.

The use of 'keepsake ultrasound' has generated considerable anxiety. A notable aspect of this anxiety is its prevalence in policy documents, in conjunction with its absence from the ethics literature. The *medical* use of foetal ultrasound has elicited critical commentary from bioethicists among others (Antiel 2012; Overall 2013; Shildrick 2015; Stephenson et al. 2016), but the *non-medical* use of foetal ultrasound seems to elicit ethical concern from a different group of stakeholders—policy-makers and healthcare providers themselves.

In 2010, the UK's Health Protection Agency issued a warning about the increasing popularity of keepsake ultrasound, noting that many healthcare agencies advise against it and regard it as ethically problematic (Public Health England 2010). Likewise, the US Food and Drug Administration warns patients against keepsake ultrasound. It argues that ultrasound should be carried out only 'when there is a medical need, based on a prescription, and performed by appropriately-trained operators' (U.S. Food and Drug Administration 2015).

As we have observed, despite the wealth of policy and regulatory documents, there are relatively few papers in the academic literature focused specifically on the ethical implications of keepsake ultrasound. However, one notable exception is a paper published in Nursing Ethics in 2009 by Leung and Pang. In this paper, the authors analyse the ethical acceptability of keepsake ultrasound. They note that medical guidelines show a high level of consensus that non-medical ultrasound is to be avoided, as well as the fact that keepsake ultrasound is typically undertaken in a commercial rather than a medical setting. Leung and Pang also observe that there is an 'absence of scientifically proven physical harm' (2009: 637) associated with the practice, and suggest that this has increased the tendency of businesses to offer the service. Another key concern is the fact that people are ill-informed about foetal ultrasound generally and what it can achieve. Their conclusion is that keepsake ultrasound is 'ethically unjustifiable' (Leung and Pang 2009: 637). Leung and Pang's analysis thus concords with the advisory guidelines and attempts to substantiate the ethical concerns that are mentioned but not explored in policy documents.

The Principles of Medical Ethics

Medicine is often regarded as having a special moral status, which keeps it in some senses 'insulated' from other human activities, especially from political, social or economic influences (Greaves 1979).

The demarcation of medicine and the reinforcement of its specifically moral significance emerged partly from the professionalisation of medicine that occurred through the nineteenth century. This process of professionalisation underpinned medicine's special status and cemented its power to control bodies, populations and political economies (Porter 2003; Pickstone 2000). Medicine is unusual in having its own system of ethics, over and above its codes of professional conduct. Doctors are perceived to be responsible not just for health, but also in some measure for morals, too. Accordingly, medical ethics has been a subject of study in its own right for some decades (Greaves 1979). The teaching and the study of medical ethics have thus served to set medicine apart morally from other human endeavours over the past century, notwithstanding the fact that 'ethicisation' is now a phenomenon that seems to be spreading across a number of other professions. While the claim to have special moral responsibilities is in part a natural development of the increasing social and professional status of doctors through the nineteenth and twentieth centuries, the importance of systematising ethics in medicine acquired particular urgency in the context of the historical events of the twentieth century.

After the Nuremberg trials, it became clear to the world that doctors and medical researchers had been actively involved in designing and carrying out a variety of medical experiments that treated concentration camp prisoners as disposable subjects for research (Weindling 2004; Smajdor et al. 2009). Further social and political changes during the latter half of the twentieth century, in conjunction with advances in medical science, contributed to the idea that a new discipline of medical ethics was required (Smajdor et al. 2011). The nineteenth-century conventions of the doctor–patient relationship were being questioned, and the traditional power and authority of doctors were increasingly treated as a cause for ethical concern (Jonsen 2000).

In the new paradigm, whatever the race or religion of the patient, and whatever the ideological convictions of the doctor, patients would be respected and protected by a universally applicable set of principles. The 'principlist' approach thus invests medicine and its practitioners with special power, which in turn imposes moral obligations towards *patients* that do not apply to *people* in a more general sense. The 'Four

Principles' approach to medical ethics attempts to set out a universally applicable approach to ethical questions in medicine, independent of social, cultural or religious contexts (Beauchamp and Childress 2009). Since its inception in the twentieth century, the four principles approach has become extremely influential and is now the dominant framework for medical ethics, though it has many critics (Clouser and Gert 1990).

The principles in question are:

- Respect for autonomy—allowing patients to make their own decisions,
- Beneficence—acting to benefit the patient,
- Non-maleficence—acting to avoid harming the patient,
- Justice—avoiding unjust discrimination and distributing resources fairly.

For medicine to function in accordance with these principles, it must be able to identify what pertains to it and what does not. It must distinguish patients from people, medical from non-medical objects/interventions and doctors from sales people. Given medicine's moral role, concepts, objects or practices that challenge the integrity of medicine's boundaries are not just intellectually challenging, but may be ethically threatening too. This is where PMDs such as keepsake ultrasound become problematic. In what follows, we look at the implications of keepsake ultrasound from the perspective of each of the four principles in turn.

Respect for Autonomy

Respect for autonomy has been termed the 'first among equals' of the four principles of medical ethics. It is generally held to entail that patients participate in the decision-making process, engaging in deliberation with the doctor, drawing on the doctor's expertise and opinion, but ultimately making their own choices (Gillon 2003). One of the first questions relating to PMDs' ethical impact should thus be to determine whether they tend to enhance or diminish patients' autonomy. As we have suggested, however, the moral duty of the doctor to respect patient autonomy relies on a clear framework within which the doctor–patient relationship is constructed. Doctors do not walk around respecting *everyone's* autonomy. It is not part of their moral obligation to do so. Because of this, defining when and in what circumstances a person is or becomes a patient is crucial.

If we construe the users of keepsake ultrasound as *patients*, the availability of this additional option appears to enhance autonomy in some respects. People can be 'introduced' to their babies in an informal setting and can use the images or videos in any way that suits their inclinations (Window to the Womb 2016). However, as we have seen, those who have commented on the ethics of keepsake ultrasound do not embrace it as an autonomy-enhancing phenomenon. Rather, it appears that the availability of keepsake ultrasound as a PMD is considered ethically threatening. Why is this? Part of the answer lies in the destabilising potential of PMDs and their impact on the doctor–patient relationship. In the days before the professionalisation of medicine, it would have made little sense to think about PMDs in terms of their impact on patients' autonomy. Medical devices and remedies were bought and sold and used in the same way as other products (Porter 2003).

The primary ethical framework of the marketplace is 'caveat emptor', i.e. 'buyer beware'. People would have had to turn a sceptical eye on the goods and services on offer as they navigated between the mountebanks and charlatans, quacks and marketplace healers, purveyors of pills, spells, prayers, unguents, artefacts and miracle cures that were available at the time (Porter 1989). The point is that where remedies were purchased in the marketplace along with other household supplies, no special category of *patient autonomy* was required, since buyers were expected to turn the same critical faculties and scepticism to medical products and claims as they did to other items. It is only with the professionalisation of medicine that the special moral category of *patient* begins to emerge. Only once this category is crystallised does the moral framework of respect for autonomy start to function.

When the problem is construed in this way, it becomes easier to see why keepsake ultrasound is morally threatening. If people can access and use PMDs such as keepsake ultrasound without the control or protection of medical institutions per se, they become more like consumers than patients. Doctors have a special moral obligation to respect the autonomy of their patients through the provision of clear and accurate information. Consumers are not protected by this kind of framework. Part of the concern over commodification of medicine relates to a fear, expressed by Leung and Pang, Pellegrino and many others, that people do not adequately understand the risks of medicine. They lack the education and training to interpret medical evidence and rely on doctors to undertake this for them.

It is this that makes respect for patient autonomy so important. Outside the carefully regulated medical world, it seems that people are at the mercy of those who stand to profit from their ignorance and vulnerability. People accessing keepsake ultrasound are likely to be informed partly by what they read on the Internet (Stöckl 2013). The public's use of Internet sources for medical information has been highlighted as a pressing problem for some years. Writing in 2001, Parker et al. observed that one of the commonest reasons people gave for using the internet was to find out information about their health. With this easily accessible resource so widely available, the role of medical professionals as 'gateways to information' has been eroded. Parker and Gray lament that health-related information will no longer respect boundaries (Parker and Gray 2001).

Some might argue that this state of affairs, far from posing an ethical problem, represents a positive advance in patient autonomy. If people no longer have to rely on doctors as the sole providers of medical information, they can gain more independence, assume more responsibility and be more autonomous. But access to information, Leung and Pang suggest, is only valuable if the information is trustworthy. Parker et al. suggest that medical data accessed online is likely to be skewed towards the particular biases of those who produce it. Specifically, much of the material that people find on the Internet is likely to be *marketing* information, and sellers do not assume the same special moral codes and responsibilities that doctors do (Lloyd, Lupton, and Donaldson 1991). Accessing medical information on the Internet is therefore often regarded as ethically worrying rather than as a welcome expansion of patient autonomy.

The implication of these arguments seems to be that information provided by bona fide healthcare professionals is pure of self-interest, devoid of bias and impervious to error. Therefore, patients can trust it implicitly, with no need for the kind of critical evaluation or scepticism that they might apply in other areas. This is precisely what has changed since the development of medical ethics and professionalised medicine. Patients can be passive under the protection of the morally trustworthy doctor in ways that they cannot be as consumers. Of course, medicine's claims to accuracy, purity and objectivity are all things that can and perhaps should be queried. Additionally, it might be argued that it is specifically the expectation of blind trust and vulnerability that renders the *medical* marketplace problematic. Some authors take it for granted that people approach their doctors with innocent faith and that this—although appropriate and necessary for medicine—is dangerous in the consumer domain. If we are genuinely concerned about patients' autonomy, their ability to protect themselves and make sensible decisions, perhaps it is this expectation of blind faith that is the problem.

But is this misguided? For Pellegrino, the role of the doctor is morally special precisely because of the power imbalance between doctors and patients (Pellegrino 1999). Patients are typically regarded as *inherently vulnerable* because they are sick and suffering (Turner 2010). Inequality is implicit in the doctor–patient relationship (Childress and Siegler 1984; Chervenak and McCullough 2011). A woman attending a medical ultrasound appointment thus has in some senses a different moral status from one who uses the Internet to book a keepsake ultrasound in order to frame the image for her mantelpiece. The former's vulnerability imposes a moral duty on the doctor not to abuse his or her power over the patient—that is, *to respect her autonomy*. Yet, the latter is also vulnerable in a different way. She is not *sick*. But she is vulnerable, on Leung and Pang's view, because she probably cannot understand and certainly should not necessarily trust the marketing information she finds online.

It might seem that this is a damning indictment not just of the commodification of medicine, but of the marketplace more generally. If consumers cannot trust information related to the purchases they make because of the self-interest of the providers of that information, they are in a bad situation in all their consumer activities. Yet, we do not see such anxietyin non-medical areas of consumer activity. This is surely not because people who are unable to understand medical information become somehow more intelligent when they are buying houses, cars, holidays or insurance, rather than health care. Rather, consumers are *expected* to be knowledgeable, to undertake research, in ways that patients are not. Indeed, the status of the consumer conveys a certain sort of power ('spending power' or 'consumer power'). This might be thought to arise from a more or less independent exercise of one's critical faculties, involving calculation not just of cost and risk, but also of the trustworthiness and bias of various sources of information.

Those who argue strongly for a clear demarcation between medicine and marketplace and between patient and consumer wish to ensure that the kind of critical evaluation employed in consumer decisions does not contaminate anything associated with medicine. Rather than arguing for better, more reliable information, so that people *can* understand and believe what they are told, Leung and Pang, and the various regulatory bodies, urge people to eschew the keepsake ultrasound altogether—to keep medicine in the clinic where it belongs. However, there is a somewhat ironic aspect to this ethical anxiety about the untrustworthiness of consumer information and the incapacity of ordinary people to make sense of medical information, in the sense that medical professionals themselves are not immune to error.

Leung and Pang discuss a number of studies that reveal clinicians' lack of understanding about medical foetal ultrasound. They describe this as 'discouraging'. From an ethical perspective, it may be more than simply discouraging. Patients' consent is not ethically valid if it is based on false information. It is not surprising that the medical provision of foetal ultrasound is thought to be poorly understood by patients who undergo scans (Harris 2004; Palmer 2009; Kohut et al. 2002; Chervenak and McCullough 2011) given that their information is being supplied by professionals who *also* lack understanding.

Thus, it appears that while keepsake ultrasound offers more choices to consumers to use the procedure in ways that suit their own interests, it is not straightforward to construe this as enhancing autonomy. The wish of the medical establishment to contain foetal ultrasound so that people can *only* access it as patientspoint towards two underlying concerns: first, to keep the distinction between patient and consumer clear; and second, to ensure that as *patients*, people rely with implicit trust on information supplied by medical professionals.

Beneficence

Beneficence—doing *good*—encapsulates what many people regard as the essence of medicine. There is ongoing debate as to the role of the doctor, but many would argue that doctors are more than just servants, mechanics, advisors or suppliers (Spiro et al. 1993). Rather, their unique and special role is to help people, to cure disease, to relieve distress and suffering, prolong lives and improve health. In short, medicine is morally special because *beneficence* is a part of it in a way that is not usually expected of other professions (Pellegrino 1999). As we have suggested, the link between medical need and healing is problematic in the case of many PMDs. Medical justification for keepsake ultrasound is tenuous or non-existent, and therefore, it cannot easily be construed as being 'beneficial' in a strictly medical sense. Rather, the benefit of the keepsake ultrasound is contingent on whatever the consumer's wishes and values may be.

However, as we have shown, maintaining the distinction between medical and non-medical is particularly troublesome in the case of keepsake ultrasound. Indeed, much of the language used in the medical sphere to explain and justify the *need* for ultrasound seems to mirror the kind of subjective value-based language one might find in the marketplace. Foetal ultrasound is often described as offering a chance to 'bond' with the baby. The NHS website states '[f]or many women, ultrasound scans are the highlight of pregnancy. It's very exciting to 'see' your baby in the womb, often moving his or her hands and legs' (National Health Service 2015). Of course, the NHS does not provide scans just for the excitement or to provide a 'highlight'. The scans are intended to identify problems with the foetus and have become a routine part of the medical management of pregnancy, so much so that it is reported that women often do not realise that they have the right to refuse to undergo them (Kohut et al. 2002). Interestingly, an American website underplays the need for ultrasound scans at all in pregnancy, unless there is a specific reason to believe there is a problem (American Pregnancy Association 2016). It is worth noting, of course, that in the USA each ultrasound scan will cost the insurer some money. Therefore, patients and insurers may be less eager to regard scans as an integral part of any pregnancy. In contrast, in a publicly funded health system such as the UK National Health Service, the costs are far more opaque to patients and often to practitioners themselves. Arguably, in the NHS, the routine nature of the scans in conjunction with lack of immediate involvement in the costs means that patients and providers alike may lose perspective of the need-based justification (if any) for the procedure.

Since the medical justification for routine foetal ultrasound is already somewhat unclear, the difficulty in maintaining a crisp boundary between medical and non-medical use is not surprising. As Leung and Pang note, many of the clinicians themselves who provide foetal ultrasound in the medical setting are uncertain as to its clinical benefits. In some senses, the difficulties relating to keepsake ultrasound can be seen as a symptom of a broader problem in the evolution of the concept of 'best interests'. As individual values and concerns have become more prominent in medical decision-making, the concept of best interests has become malleable. UK law requires best interest decisions, which are taken in the event that the patient lacks capacity to decide for him/herself, to incorporate the patient's own known wishes and values. Thus, subjectivity has crept into this domain. As we can see, this infiltration of subjectivity is particularly evident in foetal ultrasound. Patients are led to understand that their excitement and joy at seeing their baby are part of the point of the medical procedure. This in turn makes it difficult to identify clearly which instances of ultrasound are 'needed', and hence, authentically medical, and which are not.

PMDs may exacerbate this threat to doctors' special ability to determine people's best interests. If, after all, best interests are subjective in the way that colour preferences or lifestyle choices are, there seems no reason to consult a doctor. When a woman decides to get a keepsake ultrasound for the sake of the pleasure it will give her, it might seem odd to ask the doctor's advice any more than she would ask about what to watch on TV or whether to get a new haircut. While PMDs are unlikely to eliminate the concept of best interests, they certainly raise further questions about whether the user's perception of what is good for them should match that of the medical professional.

Non-maleficence

Non-maleficence is sometimes regarded as the simplest ethical principle to which doctors should adhere. It features in the Hippocratic Oath and reappears in the common phrase 'primum non nocere': first, do no harm. The importance of this principle stems largely from the recognition that those same skills that allow a doctor to improve a patient's health or well-being can in themselves cause damage, pain or sickness. The question of harm is also raised by innovation and research in medicine, which is extraordinarily closely regulated in comparison with other areas of research. Yet, the injunction 'first do no harm' is too extreme. If this really were a doctor's first and primary obligation, he or she would not be able to do anything at all. No medical procedure is entirely without risk. A vaccination causes harm by puncturing the skin; even screening may cause harm in the form of anxiety, or a false-positive result. For this reason, it is clear that non-maleficence cannot function as medicine's primary ethical principle despite the common assumption that it does. Rather, it serves as a balance against beneficence. Beneficence is an active principle; it calls for doctors to intervene to benefit their patients. Non-maleficence is a passive and cautionary principle that reminds doctors to think about the harm they may cause by intervening.

Non-maleficence might seem to be the most obvious principle that is likely to be engaged by the use of PMDs. Although PMDs may pose difficulties in classification (whether medical or non-medical), it might be thought that this should not matter, provided that they do not in fact pose significant harm to users. However, even answering this question is not straightforward. Increasingly in recent years, it has become apparent that there is a diversity of ways in which people interpret what is good or bad for them. This has always been true in the 'recreational' world, where people smoke, drink and take drugs, drive dangerous cars and participate in risky sports. However, it is also increasingly true in medicine. This has made it much more difficult to apply the principle of non-maleficence in a consistent way or to expect medicine to have objective answers as to how it applies. People have sought to use reproductive technology to conceive deaf children (Häyry 2004); others have sought to have healthy limbs amputated (Tomasini 2006). The distinction between circumcision in males (Darby 2013) and female genital mutilation (Earp 2015) is another instance of such disputes. In all these examples, the interplay between subjective values and the objectivity of harm, disease or damage leads to tension. Protecting patients from risk or harm may be unwelcome if the things they are protected from are things that they themselves regard as beneficial.

Leung and Pang and Pellegrino fear that if medicine is commodified and accessed through the marketplace, the patient/consumer will be at risk since sellers do not abide by the same special moral codes and responsibilities that doctors do. Not all would concur with this, however. Consumers do benefit from stringent protection and regulatory restrictions in today's liberal democracies. It is false to suppose that a market in which one can buy medical devices is by necessity dangerous, burdensome or untrustworthy (Bessell et al. 2003). Yet even if one accepts this, it remains the fact that *medical* products and interventions are stringently tested for safety in ways that non-medical items may not be. The language pertaining to keepsake ultrasound is a fascinating illustration of this. Ultrasound has not been tested for use in non-medical settings or for non-medical purposes. It has been rigorously tested for *medical* use only. It is this that is emphasised in the policy documents and guidelines. Outside the medical setting, who knows what dangers and harms might arise from ultrasound?

The guarantee of medical safety is a product of the regulatory system. If an item has not passed through this system, its safety is deemed to be unknown. Some of these issues were illustrated in the Poly Implant Prostheses scandal (O'Dowd 2012). It emerged that 'industrial' rather than 'medical' grade silicone had been used in breast implants. Like keepsake ultrasound, breast implants—PIP or otherwise—are often paid for by consumers and are sought by people who do not necessarily have a strictly medical need for them. The patient researches, chooses and pays for her preferred procedure and practitioner; already this is a weakening of the boundaries of medicine, as evidenced by the shades of moral opprobrium that attach to women who seek this kind of intervention. The risks that are deemed acceptable in orthodox medicine become excessive and unpalatable when patients seek out treatment for themselves.

The PIP scandal highlighted the dilemma that emerges when the borders between medical and non-medical materials are breached. Where non-medical materials infiltrate medical practice, as in the case of PIP implants, they may be perceived as dirty, polluted and harmful (O'Dowd 2012). Some experts advised the urgent removal of every PIP implant, irrespective of problematic symptoms (Dieterich et al. 2013). This would of course involve all the usual risks of surgery, in order to obviate a danger whose primary characteristic at this stage was simply a question of mis-categorisation. The scandal was not specifically that the implants were known to be *dangerous* but that they were not *medical*. The difference between industrial and medical grade silicon is not necessarily to be found in the composition of the material itself, but is a product of the regulatory process that helps to demarcate certain things as belonging to medicine. When objects or procedures cross these boundaries, it seems in some senses to *generate* risk.

Likewise, the difference between medical and keepsake ultrasound is not to be found in the equipment, the process or the personnel involved. These may be identical in each case, but extra risk is apparently generated by the symbolic difference in *purpose.* The FDA in particular highlights the risks of keepsake ultrasound. Of course, if ultrasound is risky per se, it is also risky when used routinely for screening during pregnancy. However, as we have shown, a different status pertains to risks encountered within the clinical setting from those experienced by non-medical users. Keepsake ultrasound is a particularly compelling example here, because unlike many other medical products, procedures or devices, ultrasound is described in at least one medical setting as having '*no known risks*' (National Health Service 2015). Again therefore it appears that risks are *generated* in warnings such as that issued by the FDA. Though ultrasound is not usually deemed risky, it becomes dangerous when it crosses the boundary between medicinal and recreational use.

In the context of PMDs more generally, it might seem reasonable to ask how can we be sure that those who are working to meet market rather than medical demands will create devices that are safe and reliable (Halperin et al. 2008). The marketing claims associated with PMDs could be false or overblown as suppliers attempt to persuade consumers to buy their products. In the context of keepsake ultrasound, however, these questions seem less pertinent because of the fact that the procedure is so widely acknowledged to be either risk-free or extremely low risk. A peculiar feature of Leung and Pang's paper is their oddly wistful acknowledgement that the low risk nature of ultrasound itself makes life hard for those who wish to restrict the proliferation of keepsake ultrasound.

The fact that unknown dangers and risk-related rhetoric are marshalled to urge the public to avoid keepsake ultrasound thus indicates that the dangers involved in the crossing of medical and non-medical boundariescan be largely symbolic. The question of whether specifically medical harms are intrinsically more dangerous than other types of harm is key here. Do patients need to be protected from the risks of PMDs such as keepsake ultrasoundbecause they are properly speaking 'medical', because they are *harmful* or because they are *medically harmful?* We are encouraged to see them as risky, unknown, dangerous or harmful only when used outside the medical setting. Salter et al. discuss a related issue in the context of stem cell research (Salter et al. 2015). Some innovative stem cell treatments are marketed to the public, but this tends to be highly controversial, especially among the scientific and medical community. There is an assumption that the public are vulnerable and need protection through the creation of more effective regulatory frameworks. Yet, as Salter et al. note, the increasing numbers of consumers seeking stem cell therapies seem to challenge the idea that this relationship can easily be managed. It also perhaps raises questions about how far, if at all, these supposedly vulnerable and ignorant consumers *want* to be managed (Salter et al. 2015). According to Salter and colleagues, there is a schism in stem cell research between those who adhere rigidly to medical norms of innovation and research and those who adopt a more dynamic and responsive approach. The latter are regarded with suspicion by the former. The two exemplify very different attitudes towards the public. The medical perspective views public as passive consumers of the products that researchers develop and then tell them they need. The other approach is to regard the public as active and engaged, participating in generating information and data, and setting the research agenda.

As we have shown, the presumptive passivity of patients is deeply embedded in the doctor–patient relationship as construed in the dominant approach to medical ethics. This generates the ongoing cycle of tension between autonomy, beneficence and non-maleficence, as medicine tries to maintain its role of protecting and benefiting patients, sometimes by restricting their options. For Salter et al., it seems that the prospective breakdown of the traditional doctor–patient relationship could be perceived as a positive development, which would re-invigorate and re-empower the erstwhile patient as a consumer. Whatever one's perspective on the desirability of this, it seems plausible that PMDs could feed into this transformative process.

Justice

The inclusion of justice among the principles of medical ethics reflects the degree to which medicine is no longer an interaction between doctor and patient but between populations and systems. Health systems are hugely complex institutions. In Western societies, the way in which health care is managed represents the social and political convictions of the state. Whether health care is state-provided or not, it is inescapably ideological. Publicly funded healthcare systems aim to abolish or at least diminish the degree to which inequalities in socio-economic status impinge on people's health. Our societies include people who are more and less powerful and privileged, but—in theory at least—their medical needs and their treatment transcend these boundaries so that no patient's need is deemed less important than another's, and no patient, however powerful, receives preferential treatment. It is an interesting question why *medical equality* is such a highly prized ideal in societies that accept or even welcome other sorts of inequality.

But whatever the answer to this question, this elevation of medical equality above other aspects of equality leads inescapably to contested claims about what is or is not to be deemed medical. Those interventions that the health service does *not* provide are subject to all the vicissitudes of unequal societies. In a publicly funded healthcare system such as the NHS, there is a limited budget. At its crudest level, this means that choosing to spend money on one particular patient—or even one particular condition—will mean there may be less to spend on another. We cannot provide all treatments that each patient may want or need. Because of this, we need to find ways of prioritising patients. In the NHS and similar systems, the first step is to establish clinical need.

A ruptured appendix is a paradigmatic example of the clinical need. The patient will be in pain, and if they do not receive medical attention quickly, they will die. The concept of need used in this way seems to have a certain purity. Appendicitis can affect anyone. Age, race, sexuality, financial status and nationality have little impact on one's prognosis, except insofar as they may affect one's ability to access treatment, and of course it is this—ability to access treatment—that a publicly funded healthcare system seeks to equalise. While subjectivity of values preferences and interpretations of the good are a problem in many areas of medicine, the appendix example perhaps comes closest to an objective instance of medical need independent of subjective factors. Accordingly, the provision of treatment is not contested in a publicly funded healthcare system for this kind of acute illness. But with the increasing availability of medical technology, there is more scope for people to seek medical interventions that are *not* so clearly needed. PMDs feed into this proliferation and its associated pressure on needs-based healthcare systems.

Those who access keepsake ultrasound outside the routine health service provision would not have to do so if the health services would provide as many scans as they wanted. But the NHS only provides treatment that is deemed to be 'medically required'. In this context, it is *not* the patient's personal values and preferences that dictate medical need, but medical expertise and orthodoxy. Similar reasoning governs access to cosmetic surgery. While any person may feel that they could benefit from a cosmetic procedure, only people whose wish has been medically sanctioned will be able to do so. The sanction may come from the medical analysis that shows, e.g. large breasts causing back pain, or it may arise from verification that the patient is experiencing severe psychological distress that could be alleviated by the intervention.

Already here the fault lines are perceptible. Some women have access to publicly funded cosmetic surgery without having to fulfil these criteria. A small percentage of PIP implants were provided by the NHS, for women who were deemed to *need* them, as opposed to those who merely wanted them. The women involved had had cancer and were having reconstructive surgery. A different status was given to these women's wish to change the look of their bodies, from the wish of the women who were seeking surgery without having had cancer. Yet, in both cases, the surgery imposed risks, was undertaken for cosmetic reasons and had no life-prolonging or disease-curing function.

It becomes difficult to know where to locate PMDs in a public health service if their *necessity* does not fit into the usual medical paradigms. If PMDs are provided by health systems, however, there has to be some kind of need-based rationale. In turn, there has to be a conceptual link between health needs and disease, which calls for a theory of health and illness. Such theories are surprisingly absent from policy documents and even from the ethics literature. The nature and existence of medical need and disease have largely been assumed to be self-evident. Without a clear understanding of this, difficulties in categorising PMDs and their place in a publicly funded health system are likely to arise. If PMDs are not available through the health services, it will be much harder to subject them to medical control. If they *are* available from the health service, it will be necessary to demonstrate how they meet specifically health needs.

The PIP scandal mentioned above also exemplified this tension between concepts of clinical need. Many women and doctors assumed that the 'tainted' implants should be removed. However, there were feelings among some commentators that the NHS should not have to pay for the removal of those who had had implants fitted privately. Since these women had chosen to undergo surgery, they did not *need* it, and therefore, their claim for further medical treatment to have them removed became contaminated, as it were, with the market flavour of their initial choice. It was implicit in many of the media reports that these women were culpable in some way. Blame was also cast on the clinics which had performed the surgery. Again, implicitly, those clinics that operated on a market basis, i.e. providing surgical interventions for money rather than based on need, were presented as being morally dubious.

Another focus of tension in this context is IVF. Those who argue strongly for the provision of IVF in a publicly funded health service often emphasise that infertility is a *disease* like any other (Practice Committee of the American Society for Reproductive Medicine 2013). The stakes are high in this kind of dispute. In jurisdictions where IVF is not provided, the socio-economic inequalities that affect other aspects of life become absorbed into the quasi-medical setting of fertility treatment. Thus, more affluent patients can afford services and interventions that other patients cannot. This brings pressure to bear on the ideological equality of medical need and medical treatment. In the context of IVF, there are many accessories and adjuncts to treatment that patients can use as PMDs—for example, apps to tell women when they are ovulating. As these become more prevalent, the effort to retain an ideological equality between human beings in terms of medical need and medical treatment becomes more and more difficult. The rich and powerful can use their resources to obtain what they seek. But the restrictions that designate certain items as being 'non-medical' or certain procedures such as IVF as being of lower medical priority impact more significantly on people whose spending power is limited. In the context of keepsake ultrasound, perhaps the most extreme example is that of the super-rich who are willing and able to take the step of buying an ultrasound machine for their personal use during their pregnancy.

Conclusion

There are already many different types of PMD, and it is likely that this variation will proliferate over time. This can make it difficult to identify over-arching themes and impacts that pertain to all PMDs, given that they can perform such different functions and respond to different conceptions of need. Nevertheless, our analysis of keepsake ultrasound as an example of a PMD (and the medical response to this) reveals an interwoven set of ethical concerns and anxieties that in many cases reflect those which arise in the context of other PMDs. The most pressing problem is the question of how and where to draw the boundaries of medicine. This is not just a question of epistemology but of morality, justice and power.

Greaves describes the nineteenth-century idea of medicine as being characterised by the reification of what he calls the unifactorial disease model (Greaves 1979). He differentiates between 'areas of life which are legitimately medical' and those which are not (Greaves 1979, p. 29). Thus, he presupposes at some level an objective truth to the question of medicine's appropriate domain, which, he believes, is often transgressed and under-theorised. However, as we have suggested, one can also see medicine's 'appropriate' domain as something whose boundaries are in constant flux; that what is authentically or legitimately medical is a matter of ongoing negotiation rather than factual enquiry.

Pellegrino notes that medicine itself seems to lose something of its special moral status when patients become consumers (Pellegrino 1999). Leung and Pang observe, with specific regard to keepsake ultrasound, that it represents a 'commoditised' sort of medicine (Leung and Pang 2009). These are clearly loaded terms. But they raise the question of exactly why it is that to access 'medical' products or interventions as a consumer rather than as a patient might be morally troublesome. If Pellegrino is right that medicine loses some of its moral authority in this scenario, we still face the problem of why medicine *should* have moral authority, or at the very least, why we should care whether it does or not.

Kirmayer argues that healing happens within a metaphorical logic of transformation which promises wholeness, balance and well-being (Kirmayer 2004). Yet, modern evidence-based medicine and modern healthcare systems with their time and cash constraints cannot always offer this wholeness and balance. Accordingly, alternative medicine may be successful precisely because it focuses on these aspects of the healing ritual which orthodox medicine frequently lacks. PMDs, meanwhile, exemplify aspects of both alternative and orthodox medicine, as well as elements of market forces and consumer choice, opening up a new field of contention as to medicine's proper role and boundaries. They upset the 'healing alliance' since the curation of data, the transformation of data into a diagnosis and the subsequent ritual of healing are no longer contained within a single medical environment to which they metaphorically belong (Kirmayer 2004). This ultimately renders medicine itself vulnerable. How can it protect its leaky boundaries? PMDs such as keepsake ultrasound expose these fault lines. If they facilitate the transition from patients to health consumers, then they may serve to accelerate the erosion of medicine's moral specialness.

This is regarded by opponents of keepsake ultrasound as something to be fought against. Those who adhere to a particular ideology of the high purpose and moral import of medicine are likely to agree. However, as we have shown, the high moral status of medicine itself and its ethical framework are not themselves immune from criticism; therefore, it is possible to perceive the development of PMDs such as keepsake ultrasound as posing a healthy challenge to existing norms and orthodoxies in medicine.

References

American Pregnancy Association. (2016). *Ultrasound: Sonogram.* Available at http://americanpregnancy.org/prenatal-testing/ultrasound. Accessed May 12, 2016.

Antiel, R. (2012). Ethical challenges in the new world of maternal–fetal surgery. *Seminars in Perinatology, 40*(4), 227–233.

Beauchamp, T., & Childress, J. (2009). *Principles of biomedical ethics.* Oxford: Oxford University Press.

Bessell, T., Anderson, J., Silagy, C., Sansom, L., & Hiller, J. (2003). Surfing, self-medicating and safety: Buying non-prescription and complementary medicines via the internet. *Quality and Safety in Health Care, 12*(2), 88–92.

Chervenak, F., & McCullough, L. (2011). Ethics in obstetric ultrasound: The past 25 years in perspective. *Donald School Journal of Ultrasound in Obstetrics and Gynecology, 5*(2), 79–84.

Childress, J., & Siegler, M. (1984). Metaphors and models of doctor-patient relationships: Their implications for autonomy. *Theoretical Medicine, 5*(1), 17.

Clouser, K., Danner, P., & Gert, B. (1990). A critique of principlism. *Journal of Medicine and Philosophy, 15*(2), 219–236.

Darby, R. (2013). The child's right to an open future: Is the principle applicable to non-therapeutic circumcision? *Journal of Medical Ethics, 39*(7), 463–468.

Dieterich, M., Stubert, J., Stachs, A., Radke, A., Reimer, T., & Gerber, B. (2013). Ruptured poly-implant protheses breast implant after aesthetic breast augmentation: Diagnosis, case management, and histologic evaluation. *Aesthetic Plastic Surgery, 37*(1), 91–94.

Earp, B. (2015). Do the benefits of male circumcision outweigh the risks? A critique of the proposed CDC guidelines. *Frontiers in Pediatrics, 3*(18). doi: 10.3389/fped.2015.00018.

Gillon, R. (2003). Ethics needs principles—Four can encompass the rest—And respect for autonomy should be "first among equals". *Journal of Medical Ethics, 29*(5), 307–312.

Greaves, D. (1979). What is medicine?: Towards a philosophical approach. *Journal of Medical Ethics, 5,* 29–32.

Halperin, D., Kohno, T., Heydt-Benjamin, T., Fu, K., & Maisel, W. (2008). Security and privacy for implantable medical devices. *Pervasive Computing, IEEE, 7*(1), 30–39.

Harris, J. (2004). Before birth–after death. *Journal of Medical Ethics, 30*(5), 425.

Häyry, M. (2004). There is a difference between selecting a deaf embryo and deafening a hearing child. *Journal of Medical Ethics, 30*(5), 510–512.

Jonsen, A. (2000). *A short history of medical ethics.* New York, Oxford: Oxford University Press.

Kirmayer, L. (2004). The cultural diversity of healing: Meaning, metaphor and mechanism. *British Medical Bulletin, 69*(1), 33–48.

Kohut, R., Dewey, D., & Love, E. (2002). Women's knowledge of prenatal ultrasound and informed choice. *Journal of Genetic Counseling, 11*(4), 265–276.

Leung, J., & Pang, S. (2009). Ethical analysis of non-medical fetal ultrasound. *Nursing Ethics, 16*(5), 637–646.

Lloyd, P., Lupton, D., & Donaldson, C. (1991). Consumerism in the health care setting: An exploratory study of factors underlying the selection and evaluation of primary medical services. *Australian Journal of Public Health, 15*(3), 194–201.

National Health Service. (2015). Ultrasound scan. Available online at: http://www.nhs.uk/conditions/Ultrasound-scan/Pages/Introduction.aspx. Accessed January 13, 2016.

O'Dowd, A. (2012). Women have had "harrowing" experiences over PIP implants scandal. *British Medical Journal, 345,* e4560.

Overall, C. (2013). *Ethics and human reproduction: A feminist analysis.* London: Routledge.

Palmer, J. (2009). The placental body in 4D: Everyday practices of non-diagnostic sonography. *Feminist Review, 93*(1), 64–80.

Parker, M., & Gray, M. (2001). What is the role of clinical ethics support in the era of e-medicine? *Journal of Medical Ethics, 27*(suppl1), i33–i35.

Pellegrino, E. (1999). The commodification of medical and health care: The moral consequences of a paradigm shift from a professional to a market ethic. *Journal of Medical Philosophy, 24*(3), 243–266.

Pickstone, J. (2000). Production, community and consumption: The political economy of twentieth-century medicine. In R. Cooter & J. Pickstone (Eds.), *Medicine in the 20th century* (pp. 1–21). Australia: Harwood Academic Publishers.

Porter, R. (1989). *Health for sale: Quackery in England, 1660–1850.* Manchester: Manchester University Press.

Porter, R. (2003). *Quacks: Fakers & charlatans in medicine.* Stroud: Tempus.

Practice Committee of the American Society for Reproductive Medicine. (2013). Definitions of sterility and recurrent pregnancy loss: A committee opinion. *Fertility and Sterility, 99*(1), 63.

Public Health England. (2010). Response to Agnir Report. Available online at https://www.gov.uk/government/publications/ultrasound-and-infrasound-hpa-response-to-agnir-report-rce-14/ultrasound-and-infrasound-hpa-response-to-agnir-report-rce-14. Accessed August 08, 2016.

Roberts, J., Griffiths, F., Verran, A., & Ayre, C. (2015). Why do women seek ultrasound scans from commercial providers during pregnancy? *Sociology of Health & Illness, 37*(4), 594–609.

Salter, B., Zhou, Y., & Datta, S. (2015). Hegemony in the marketplace of biomedical innovation: Consumer demand and stem cell science. *Social Science and Medicine, 131,* 156–163.

Shildrick, M. (2015). *Leaky bodies and boundaries: Feminism, postmodernism and (Bio) ethics.* London: Routledge.

Smajdor, A., Sydes, M. R., Gelling, L., & Wilkinson, M. (2009). Applying for ethical approval for research in the United Kingdom. *British Medical Journal. 16.* 339.

Smajdor, A., Stöckl, A., & Salter, C. (2011). The limits of empathy: Problems in medical education and practice. *Journal of Medical Ethics, 37,* 380–383.

Spiro, H., McCrea Curnen, M., Peschel, E., & St James, D. (Eds.). (1993). *Empathy and the Practice of Medicine. Beyond pills and the scalpel.* New Haven and London: Yale University.

Stephenson, N., McLeod, K., & Mills, C. (2016). Ambiguous encounters, uncertain foetuses: Women's experiences of obstetric ultrasound. *Feminist Review, 113*(1), 17–33.

Stöckl, A. (2013). The expert patient and usage of the Internet. In P. Cavanagh, S. Leinster, & S. Miles (Eds.), *The changing roles of doctors* (pp. 69–79). New York: Radcliffe Publishing.

Tomasini, F. (2006). Exploring ethical justification for self-demand amputation. *Ethics & Medicine, 22*(2), 99–115.

Turner, B. (2010). *Vulnerability and human rights.* University Park, Pennsylvania: The Pennsylvania State University Press.

U.S. Food and Drug Administration. (2015). *Avoid fetal "Keepsake" images, heartbeat monitors.* Washington: FDA.

Weindling, P. (2004). *Nazi medicine and the Nuremberg trials: From medical war trials to informed consent.* Basingstoke, Hampshire/New York: Palgrave Macmillan.

Window to the Womb. (2016). Available online at http://windowtothewomb. co.uk/. Accessed May 13, 2016.

8

Slippery Slopes and Trojan Horses: The Construction of E-Cigarettes as Risky Objects in Public Health Debate

Rebecca Lynch

Introduction

The availability and use of electronic, or 'e', cigarettes have grown extensively since 2012, and it is estimated that approximately 2.8 million people use them in the UK alone (ASH 2016). Over this time, shops devoted to selling e-cigarettes and cafes for e-cigarette use have sprung up across the UK, Internet messaging boards and social groups have been formed through the identity of being an e-cigarette user, and new language has developed around the practices of e-cigarette use, with 'e-cigs' and 'vaping' being added to the Oxford Online Dictionary in 2014. The spread and development of e-cigarettes are being undertaken both by big tobacco companies and by smaller and (at present) independent companies. Promotional material produced to market e-cigarettes differs in its emphasis. Some explicitly suggest the objects are beneficial to health

R. Lynch (✉)
London School of Hygiene and Tropical Medicine, London, UK
e-mail: Rebecca.Lynch@lshtm.ac.uk

© The Author(s) 2018
R. Lynch and C. Farrington (eds.), *Quantified Lives and Vital Data*,
Health, Technology and Society, https://doi.org/10.1057/978-1-349-95235-9_8

as an alternative to tobacco cigarettes, whereas other advertisements push cultural appeals, promoting these objects as 'cool' or glamorous, or emphasising the ability to 'vape' in a range of places where smoking would not be permitted.

This growth has attracted the attention of those working in public health, who have sought to predict what the impact of these new objects might be on the health and behaviour of the population. This has typically involved comparison of e-cigarettes with tobacco cigarettes, an association which raises the stakes for assessing their impact. The reduction in tobacco cigarette use through the introduction of higher taxes and bans on advertising, selling, and places where tobacco smoking is permitted has been seen as a success story in public health. These measures have been viewed as resulting in tobacco smoking becoming 'denormalised' (Bell et al. 2010), leading to a general cultural shift where smoking is no longer part of usually acceptable behaviour.[1] In other words, public health interventions have succeeded in stigmatising smoking (Bell et al. 2010). Despite this shift, however, there remains a concern that denormalisation does not aid those 'addicted' to tobacco, nor prevent groups of potential new smokers (usually seen as children and adolescents) from taking up tobacco (Hsu et al. 2013). How e-cigarettes may add to, or detract from, previous successes in combating tobacco use and these enduring concerns is therefore of high interest and importance to public health scientists.

Like other concerns of public health, debates on e-cigarette use revolve around the management of risk and future risk. As a new technology, debates around e-cigarettes have had to start without much evidence as to their use and impact, and to what extent these objects are themselves 'risky'. Despite this, or perhaps because of this, opinion in public health has fallen into two camps: those in favour of e-cigarettes, who view them as medical devices or treatments (e.g. Britton and Bogdanovica 2014; Etter 2013; McNeill et al. 2015; Hajek 2013; Stimson 2014), and those who are against them, viewing them as potentially harmful (e.g. Abrams 2014; De Andrade et al. 2013; Chapman 2013, 2014; Fairchild et al. 2014; Hsu et al. 2013; McKee and Capewell 2015). Those who are positive about such technology suggest that these are the most useful smoking cessation aids yet devised—a personal medical device providing a safe delivery mechanism for nicotine which can be used by a person as they would a cigarette. For those who are against e-cigarettes, these are potentially harmful objects, whose sale and use give a legitimate public presence to cigarette-like objects and to smoking-like behaviour. This, it is feared, will undo 'decades of work' by 're-normalising' smoking and encouraging people to continue, or to start, to smoke (Hsu et al. 2013). One side of the debate, therefore, believes that the impact of e-cigarettes will be that fewer people will smoke tobacco, while the other fears that more people will do so.

This chapter examines the ways in which biomedicine, in this case public health science, has sought to understand and locate e-cigarettes as a new development which may, or may not, be a personal medical device (PMD). While earlier book chapters considered the personal relationships of individual users to PMDs, this chapter looks at the impact and positioning of a possible PMD within a wider area of concern—how medical research conceptualises e-cigarettes in relation to their impact on health. As Jeanette Pols notes of the introduction of telecare, innovative technologies can see individuals rushing to declare both the positives and negatives of new devices and the impact they will have (2012). Pols makes the point, however, that new technologies can do new and unexpected things in practice, with people using these in unpredictable ways. She cites the example of the telephone becoming popular as it was used to facilitate 'the social chatter of American women, even if its designers created it to transmit the business conversations of American men' (2012, p. 18). Through her own study, it becomes clear that the telecare devices at the centre of her research—predicted to reduce professionals' workload through less contact with patients, creating care devoid of human contact—instead *increased* contact between carers and patients. These new technologies did not emerge as being cold, rational and functional in opposition to warm, comforting, human care as was initially suggested (Pols 2012). As Pols states of telecare, arguments about supposed impacts may be less of a *debate* and more *juxtapositions,* which contest '"inevitable" futures' (2012, p. 12). Indeed the two sides in the e-cigarette debate have become completely polarised, resulting in mud-slinging and divisions.

Such impassioned arguments reveal an emotional element officially banished from scientific positioning, which otherwise claims to rely on cold, hard evidence. This evidence base has often relied on randomised controlled trials (RCTs), which, Pols suggests, discipline an individual's personal and subjective knowledge. These put 'objective' knowledge in place as evidence to demonstrate the effectiveness of an intervention, leaving no (official) place for subjective positioning (Pols 2012, p. 138). However, robust RCTs take time to carry out, and the field of new technologies is fast-developing. By the time a trial has been funded and set up, the intervention technology may have moved on. An example of this can be seen in the Get Moving trial, which aimed to increase physical activity through the use of self-monitoring wristbands providing feedback data about individual activity (Cooper et al. 2015). While this was cutting-edge technology at the time of the development of the trial, by the time the trial was funded and undertaken sleeker commercial products allowing more sophisticated interaction with data (such as the Nike Fuel band and downloadable smartphone apps) had been developed and made the trial technology appear embarrassingly ugly, old and clunky (Lynch and Cohn 2015).

As well as the problems with trialling technologies that have already been superseded or made redundant by the time the trial results are published, such trials are limited in their ability to pick up nuanced aspects of the use of novel technologies, such as the new places, practices and components that accompany these, as well as changes over time and in different contexts. Even as an evidence base of the impact of e-cigarettes is built up, this is, therefore, unlikely to produce definitive results, and 'objective' evidence produced can be employed selectively and strategically, and in relation to particular audiences (Ecks 2008). Not only is it hard to generate evidence on the impact of e-cigarettes, but it is also unlikely the called-for research trials will reconcile the stances in this debate. This can be seen in responses to publications on e-cigarette use, such as the report published by Public Health England (PHE), which found positive results (Public Health England 2015; McNeill et al. 2015). This was criticised by fellow public health scientists as being:

methodologically weak, … which is made all the more perilous by the declared conflicts of interest surrounding its funding… [It] raises serious questions not only about the conclusions of the PHE report, but also about the quality of the agency's peer review process. (McKee and Capewell 2015)

That such arguments question the 'objective' nature of the evidence produced is no surprise given their origin in a framework which prioritises 'objectivity' of judgment. The 'objective' assessment, and associated positioning of objects within it, is of course how the scientific process deals with uncertainties. While there is substantial disagreement between the two sides of the e-cigarettes debate, both sides are eager to position these new and uncertain technologies somewhere within a particular frame of understanding—a positioning which relates to the predicted riskiness of these objects.

In his sociological examination of the science of public health, Kevin Dew argues that as chronic rather than infectious disease has become a greater concern for public health, risk factor epidemiology has taken a more central role (Dew 2012).[2] Connecting people to individualised risk factors which make them susceptible to disease locates the source of health and illness within the individual body and individual choices and actions, or 'behaviours'. Some behaviours are seen as particularly risky to health and therefore have become foci for public health interventions. For many public health research teams, there are four key 'health behaviours'—diet, alcohol use, level of physical activity and tobacco use. These can put individuals at greater or lesser risk of ill health, and particular objects and substances—sugar, alcohol and cigarettes for example—are associated with these behaviours as risky objects. Despite this understanding, however, risks are not neutral, and there are wider consequences for framing behaviour and objects as 'risky'. Alongside conceptualisations of risk, notions of responsibility, blame and morality also emerge, so that risky objects, and users of these objects, are also positioned positively or negatively in a moral framework. Individualistic understandings of health and personal responsibility for health fit well with the construction of risk factor epidemiology. Individual 'health behaviours', and therefore use of particular objects, are the choice (and responsibility) of individuals themselves.

Context and Framing

Situated as an anthropologist in a multi-disciplinary public health research team that sought to add to the growing evidence on the impact of e-cigarettes, my argument is drawn both from participation observation within the team and from analysis of scientific papers and commentaries produced by the scientific community which were emerging on this topic between 2013 and 2015. Through the research meetings, discussions and email exchanges I participated in (between December 2013 and September 2014) and also evident through the discourses produced more broadly within public health over this time, I observed how research scientists sought to give this new technology a value and moral positioning by placing it within a wider medical (and consequently moralising) framework. The two sides of the debate emerged and became more polarised through these discussions and over time, and this was a split we had to negotiate as researchers in interactions, collaborations and everyday research tasks. From an anthropological perspective, it also became clear that researchers on both sides were constructing e-cigarettes as particular *types* of objects which drew on similar fundamental understandings within public health. This meant that while e-cigarettes were being constructed as different objects by the two sides in the debate, these conceptualisations relied on the same understandings of objects and people, and the relationship between these.

Objects can be conceptualised as connected to, created by and interacting with other actors such as materials, people, other objects and infrastructure in a co-constituted way (Maller 2015, p. 54), and as emerging from the context they are situated within rather than existing independently 'outside' it. Practice theorists and approaches from science and technology studies suggest that objects are created or 'enacted' through practices (Mol 2002). Mol's work on atherosclerosis, for example, proposes that this disease, like other diseases and indeed like the body itself, is 'made' through the various practices undertaken by clinicians, surgeons, laboratory technicians and patients (Mol 2002). Instead of taking what Law and Singleton refer to as an 'epistemological' approach—looking at one object (or one disease, in the case of atherosclerosis) seen differently by people with different perspectives on this—this is rather an 'ontological' perspective, where different enactments of an object make different objects (Law and Singleton 2005; Mol 2002). So the work undertaken by clinicians, surgeons, laboratory technicians and patients in the example of Mol's study *make* different athersercloses, and different bodies, through their different enactments. In the context of the e-cigarettes debate therefore, this approach suggests that the fundamental difference between the two sides is not merely an epistemological distinction between different perspectives on the same object, but an ontological distinction. Through their practices, the two sides enact e-cigarettes in different ways, so that e-cigarettes are made as different objects that 'are' different things.

Rather than considering the growing evidence of e-cigarette use and impact, or trying to reconcile these positions, I instead wish to focus on how e-cigarettes are constructed as (different) objects in these public health debates. I look to move beyond the entrenched dichotomy of opinion by asking whether e-cigarettes might be considered different types of objects, over and beyond a medical device or a device masquerading as such. Presenting an alternative future for e-cigarettes, I suggest some limitations of the ways public health science constructs its objects of study and how an alternative focuses on objects in analysis may take us to different, and perhaps more productive, places.

E-cigarettes as Types of Cigarettes

For one side of the debate, e-cigarettes presented a number of potential harms. E-cigarettes might act as smoking 'cues' (2013), the increasing popularity and marketing of e-cigarettes having already resulted in an increased presence of 'cigarette-like objects, images and smoking behaviour' which may renormalise smoking (Hsu et al. 2013, p. 5). Others focused on the new role that e-cigarettes-as-medical-treatments allowed tobacco companies to take, becoming partners in health policy (Chapman 2013; De Andrade et al. 2013). In an impassioned opinion piece, Professor of Public Health Simon Chapman suggests the promotion of e-cigarettes is of great advantage to the tobacco industry as a means to keep people smoking, 'conveying to young, apprehensive would-be smokers that nicotine is a benign drug; and welcoming back lapsed smokers' (Chapman 2013, p. 3840). Suggesting that this in danger of becoming 'one of the biggest blunders of modern public health', Chapman insists that '[w]e should make none of the disastrous mistakes made with cigarettes ... We should not start by assuming they are benign items of commerce' (Chapman 2013, p. 3840). For those on this side of the debate, then, e-cigarettes were risky objects, not 'benign' objects—they were objects *masquerading* as personal medical devices.

Underpinning this argument is the notion that e-cigarettes are a *type* of cigarette. Through this construction, e-cigarettes are so similar to tobacco cigarettes that they are viewed as another version of the same kind of object. This common-sense argument was also seen in public reactions to e-cigarettes and in the rationale for banning their use in some public places. For example, in statements given by the British pub and bar chains, J.D. Wetherspoon and Fuller's Inns as to why e-cigarettes were banned in their establishments, the managing director of Fuller's Inns is quoted as telling a trade magazine that:

> For non-smoking customers, the sight of a customer using an e-cigarette is disconcerting, especially it's often hard to tell the difference between a tobacco cigarette and an e-cigarette from distance, which causes added anxiety for our guests. (*The Publican's Morning Advertiser* 2013)

As e-cigarettes so resembled tobacco cigarettes, others present might *think* or *assume* that the person was smoking tobacco, leading to some undisclosed anxiety—perhaps relating to second-hand smoke exposure, or discomfort arising from another's rule-breaking. However, this argument of 'typing' falls down in a number of areas.

Richard Klein's book on the philosophical, literary and cultural history of cigarettes (*Cigarettes Are Sublime* 1995) suggests that tobacco cigarettes are among the most significant objects of our time and a crucial integer of modernity, with their introduction to Europe coinciding with the spread of books, the development of the scientific method and increased questioning of theological positions. Cigarettes have been objects of gift and trade, portrayed in particular ways in literature, photography and film and have provided a language of acts and gestures. As newer objects, some e-cigarettes have been marketed in similar ways to cigarettes and have started to be depicted in popular culture, featuring in film and television shows where tobacco cigarettes would not permitted, such as the film 'The Tourist' (Bell and Keane 2012; De Andrade et al. 2013) or the popular UK soap opera 'Eastenders' (De Andrade et al. 2013). However, neither the experience of smoking tobacco cigarettes, nor the multitude of symbolic meanings attached to tobacco cigarettes, can be directly taken on by e-cigarettes. Klein notes for example that the act of smoking may be an act of defiance or a time for meditation or composure, opening a gap of time in everyday ordinary experience. E-cigarettes do not 'take' a similar time to consume in this way, however—a cigarette break (lasting as long as a cigarette takes to smoke) is not a similarly defined time period for an e-cigarette. As well as the self-consuming nature of tobacco cigarettes, the social act of sharing a packet does not translate to e-cigarette use, and nor are the range of designs, use of technological apparatus and wide range of flavours of e-cigarettes found in tobacco cigarettes. While a logical comparison of objects independent of context may see these objects as the same, as soon as an analytic focus is moved to situating the object within smoking practices, it becomes more difficult to assume that e-cigarettes and tobacco cigarettes will have the same pattern of use and associations.

Moreover, these discourses not only group e-cigarettes into a wider category of 'cigarettes' but also lump together a wide range of objects under this term. The category of 'e-cigarettes' actually incorporates a range of different products of varying types. While public health discussions often group these together, in marketing these products and in online user forums significant distinctions are made between various forms of e-cigarettes, such as 'vaporisers' or 'e-hookahs'. Terming all these products, 'e-cigarettes' retains and reinforces the link to tobacco cigarettes, despite the fact that only a few of these technologies closely resemble traditional cigarettes. Instead, many have obvious metal, glass and plastic components, can be bought in a range of colours, and can be modified and personalised not only in look but also by flavour, chemical mix and nicotine content. By their very nature, therefore, some types of e-cigarettes can be tailored to fit the user and user requirements—they are objects that people can form, and express, a longer-term relationship with as they personalise and refuel the same piece of equipment. The technology of e-cigarettes also requires engagement and use of different smoking paraphernalia such as chargers or refills. Again, considering these objects in context and in use moves further away from a simple comparison with tobacco cigarettes.

Inherent in the logic of this side of the argument, and again reinforcing the idea that these are the same sorts of objects as tobacco cigarettes, is the notion of the 'slippery slope' that leads individuals from one object, or substance, to another. This viewpoint suggests a single continuum of substances, with people being seen to migrate from e-cigarettes to tobacco cigarettes with relative ease. The same argument has been applied in terms of drug use, with people moving from cannabis to harder drugs along this one continuum (e.g. Kandel 2003). This assumes an inherent vulnerability with people slipping from one object to another unproblematically, and that these objects are so similar that they are interchangeable—that cannabis is in some way the same as heroin, and that vaping an e-cigarette is the same as smoking a tobacco cigarette. From a perspective that focuses on user experiences and practices, however, this is not so smooth and inevitable a move.

The use of different drugs do not involve the same actions; they have different physiological effects and different contexts and meanings. This perspective also constructs the user as passive and lacking in will, as 'addicted' and unable to escape the power of the object or substance itself. This lack of individual will in the face of such a powerful object imbues both those smoking and the drugs themselves with a form of morality: smokers are 'weak' and drugs are 'dangerous' and 'addictive'. This implied morality around addictive objects and substances, and around addicts and addiction in general (a perspective also found in discourses on obesity, e.g. Puhl and Heuer 2010), can be tied to broader cultural understandings of the importance of self-control and self-mastery as an indicator of civility (Bennett 2013): we *should* be able to control and monitor ourselves in relation to these objects, and addiction is, therefore, a failure of will. Those who are addicted have less self-control and are somehow deficient.

E-cigarettes as a Copy of the Original

For those who focus on the benefits of e-cigarettes, these are constructed as objects which could lead to the end of smoking-related disease (Hajek 2013). From this perspective, smokers will 'switch' to e-cigarettes as 'an alternative and much safer source of nicotine, as a personal lifestyle choice' (Britton and Bogdanovica 2014). As another public health professor, Jean-François Etter, points out, e-cigarettes do not need to be completely 'safe', only safer than tobacco cigarettes. This is about harm reduction, then, where alternative risks posed by different substances are weighed up to reduce risks to the individual, even if these are not removed completely. As Etter states: 'Even if some former smokers remain addicted to the nicotine delivered by e-cigarettes, this is not a public health problem because e-cigarettes have not been proved to be toxic. Thousands of former smokers are addicted to nicotine gum, and this is not a public health problem either' (Etter 2013, p. 3845). For Etter, e-cigarettes offer a 'revolution in public health' and as many smokers should be pushed into using e-cigarettes as possible (Etter 2013). These are therefore medical devices: they are only *appearing* to be a type of cigarette but in fact, they are a *copy* of a cigarette. They are not cigarettes masquerading as medical devices but are medical devices masquerading as cigarettes. They are simulants (and stimulants of course!)—they simulate the real thing, the tobacco cigarette, mimicking this but remaining a copy.

It is in the mimetic faculty of the copy that its power lies, as the anthropologist Michael Taussig states: 'The wonder of mimesis lies in the copy drawing on the character and power of the original, to the point whereby the representation may even assume that character and that power' (1993, p. xiii). Through their mimicry of tobacco cigarettes, e-cigarettes may 'seem' to be cigarettes but actually, they are quite different objects. While on the outside resembling a cigarette, they are actually delivering something else, like a Trojan horse. Through being a convincing copy, they have the potential to be subversive and useful objects in making changes to health behaviour. As a convincing simulant, this side of the argument theorises that people would find it easy to form the same relationship with a copy as they did with the original, moving away from being addicted to tobacco cigarettes to (being addicted to) e-cigarettes. Taussig's work on mimesis goes further, suggesting that not only is there a power drawn from the original in the copy, but also in the power of a copy to influence the original. He compares this to James Frazer's early anthropological understanding of sympathetic magic, or the use of powerful copies to magically affect what they are copies of (Frazer 1890). This can be seen in practices associated with 'voodoo' or other forms of magic where a lock of hair or fingernail represents a person, so that enacting magic using these bodily parts impacts on the person who has been represented. Arguments for the benefits of e-cigarettes also draw on a sort of sympathetic magic argument in suggesting that e-cigarettes have the power to impact on tobacco cigarette use—the power of the copy affects how the original is used.

Taussig developed his work from Walter Benjamin's essay 'The Work of Art in the Age of Mechanical Reproduction' (1968/1955) which raises questions about reproduction and authenticity in relation to works of art. Looking at mass reproduction, Benjamin suggests that while the original piece of art is an independent object from the copy, through the act of reproduction something is taken from the original, changing its context. At the same time, the original retains something that will always be lacking from the copy. The original's 'presence in time and space', what he terms the 'aura' of a piece of work, is absent in a reproduction. As simulants, e-cigarettes draw on the power of original cigarettes in their construction and appeal, but without the aura of cigarettes, can these ever be a replacement?

The particular aura of cigarettes has been portrayed through many cultural sources including literature, photography and film, for example in well-known glamorous photographs of Marlene Dietrich and the notion of the 'Humphrey Bogart cigarette' (Klein 1995) from which the slang term for a cigarette as a 'bogey' also developed. Klein compares the sublimity of the tobacco cigarette to creating a poem:

> inhaling the hot breath of inspiration, letting words on a page burn up in the visible air of a muted electrocution, exhaling swirling figures of desire, conducting with gestures and modulating in smoke a lyric conversation overheard. (Klein 1995, p. 51)

Klein suggests that the cigarette's bad taste and poisonousness add to their sublimity; they are somehow edgy and dangerous. While e-cigarettes are a copy of a tobacco cigarette, their materiality differs—they contain none of tobacco's poisonousness and can be inhaled in a range of non-threatening-sounding flavours, such as 'caramel mocha', 'mango mirage' and 'apple grape breeze' (flavoured liquids produced by UK Ecig Store). This makes them neither edgy nor dangerous, neither poetic nor sublime. The copy lacks the 'aura' of the original, as e-cigarettes lack the sublimity of tobacco cigarettes.

Discourses around pleasure, and certainly on sublimity, are notably missing from the debates on e-cigarette use. This is perhaps not surprising as these concepts are relatively neglected in public health more broadly. Notions of pleasure are ignored in the attempt to promote health and wider well-being, while addicts and substances are morally positioned (Coveney and Bunton 2003).[3] Benson (2010) argues that dependence on nicotine has been increasingly medicalised and viewed as a chronic condition, while Bell and Keane (2012) note that nicotine has somewhat contradictorily been understood as both a cause and treatment for cigarette addiction.[4] The role of nicotine patches and chewing gum ('good' nicotine) have been situated as forms of treatment for cigarette addiction (caused by 'bad' nicotine), reinforced through evidence of effectiveness demonstrated in research trials (Bell and Keane, *ibid.*), much as current research on e-cigarette use seeks to establish. However, Bell and Keane note that e-cigarettes have received a more hostile reception than other nicotine delivery treatments and suggest that this is because e-cigarettes challenge the distinction between nicotine as either a treatment or a harm, and therefore either 'good' or 'bad' nicotine. 'Good' nicotine should not resemble a cigarette, nor should it be connected to pleasure (Bell and Keane 2012).

Furthermore, by replacing one substance for another, public health and medical discourses could be said to be controlling which substances the public are addicted to. This can be compared to the relationship between methadone and heroin, and the UK comedian Russell Brand's argument that that methadone is merely a medicalised form of heroin, allowing the state to control the substance that the individual is addicted to as a means of controlling addiction. The nicotine within e-cigarettes remains addictive, and through medicalisation, the key difference in the promotion of e-cigarettes then becomes that it is *what* people are addicted to that is altered, rather than a removal of the addiction completely. This can be viewed as a further example of the medicalisation of everyday actions, behaviour and objects which then become subject to biomedical control (Conrad 1992), in this case meaning that government and biomedicine are able to select which substances the public are and are not allowed to become addicted to. Medicalisation justifies intervention and control, giving a foundation on which to base regulation of these products, but it does not take into account what the experience, use and material aspects of e-cigarettes may be.

E-cigarettes as Better Than the Original

A key problem with the debate on e-cigarettes is that both sides assume that they know how to conceive of these objects and establish what e-cigarettes *are*—slippery slopes or Trojan horses. But based on these assumptions, we might consider other possibilities of what an e-cigarette might be. Abrams suggests that '[i]ndependent manufacturers of e-cigarettes could compete with tobacco companies and make the cigarette obsolete, just as digital cameras made film obsolete' (Abrams 2014, p. 136). Rather than e-cigarettes being types of cigarettes or being simulants, e-cigarettes could be considered 'simulacra', the philosopher Jean Baudrillard's concept of imitations that become more 'real' or pleasurable that the real thing, which he links to postmodern culture. Baudrillard (1994/1981) suggests that postmodern society is so dependent on models and maps *of* the world that we become out of touch with the *real* world. Contemporary examples of this might include individuals experiencing events unravelling in front of them through screens as they are filmed on mobile phones, or people turning away from the action to capture themselves within an image of it in the form of a 'selfie'. Objects that are simulacra link to Baudrillard's wider concern that we have lost contact with what is 'real', with consumer society and simulacrum taking over 'reality'. Plastic surgery and breast augmentation procedures, where the fake body and breasts are viewed as more desirable, are another examples of the 'fake' becoming more 'real' than the original. Baudrillard suggests these objects are a form of 'hyper-reality'—through something becoming more real than the real, reality is abolished. Might e-cigarettes become 'even better than the real thing', more attractive than tobacco cigarettes themselves and more than a mix of tobacco cigarette and medical device?

It is possible also to argue that the e-cigarette market is already moving away from e-cigarettes being simulacra. E-cigarettes are becoming even less like tobacco cigarettes as they are being made to taste different, look different, and be more personalisable. E-cigarette development is linked to technological changes and may be limited and/or led by the technology itself. Some commentators see a new generation of e-cigarettes being developed which will cause those presently in circulation to appear old-fashioned and obsolete. New relationships are formed with new objects and there is a huge and expanding range of e-cigarettes varying not only by design and chemical ingredient but also in contexts of use. These objects, and the practices that go alongside them, are far from stable, so that the entrenched arguments held up from within public health already make little sense to many users and non-users of e-cigarettes. More to the point, perhaps, is that while public health attempts to capture a notion of what an e-cigarette 'is', such objects are not singular and fixed, and they do not exist independently of environments. If we follow Mol's argument of multiplicity, debates in public health have already 'made' e-cigarettes into (at least) two different objects through their different constructions, objects that are likely to be constructed differently again through the practices of different users.

Constructing 'Risky Objects' in Public Health

While we might know little of the impact of e-cigarette use on the general population, the ways these objects have impacted on the field of public health are more evident. E-cigarettes have become part of public health science itself—the subject of seminars, papers and policy documents, creating research groups and alliances, grants and jobs. In efforts to generate evidence, the assumptions behind the relationships between objects, people and notions of behaviour have already worked themselves into the design and conduct of behavioural interventions and evaluations, with the enactment of e-cigarettes as particular 'things' being made and remade through ongoing discourses and practices. The construction of e-cigarettes is therefore not only shaped by public health but also shapes public health itself. This highlights the key issue within this debate—that e-cigarettes, like other objects, are inevitably embedded within and co-constituted through wider environments and cannot be examined separately from these. Even as e-cigarettes are constructed in public health as static objects independent of contexts and practices, at the same time they are being further embedded within public health as objects that are dynamic and changing.

Public health science does not conceptualise objects in this dynamic way. As well as both sides of the debate constructing e-cigarettes based on tobacco cigarettes, e-cigarettes are also framed externally to their use, as static and independent objects separate from context. They are seen to have particular inherent qualities which mean that they are interchangeable with other similar objects, with e-cigarettes and tobacco cigarettes seen as a transposable 'thing'. This view of objects as separate and static is also one outside of time. As objects independent of context, they are not seen as changing over time, so that how they 'are' in the present will continue in the future. This is the key for conceptualising risk—objects need to be viewed as consistent in order to have a predictable future outcome.

However, it is not only objects that are seen as external to context but also people, and the relationship between person and object—in this case, smokers (potential, former or current) and cigarette (of whatever type)—is also constructed in a particular way. Through both sides of the argument, e-cigarettes are viewed as determining the actions resulting from their use, with e-cigarettes practices resulting from what the e-cigarette does to the person. Through this set-up, the presence of a cigarette, whether a tobacco cigarette or an e-cigarette, acts on the smoker—the smoker does not influence this object but is a 'passive' user of it. Conceptualisations of risk within public health also set up such a relationship—a one-directional connection where the object acts on the individual in a fairly consistent way, across different groups of people and different environments, through a quality inherent to the object itself.

The object is seen to act on the individual as a psychological 'cue' to the smoker to perform the action of smoking—the impact seen to be so powerful in denormalisation arguments. Smoking behaviour is therefore constructed as a cognitive practice which occurs from a smoker choosing to smoke, or being prompted to smoke by the object. Through this framing addiction is a physical dependence on a substance, which impairs the cognitive process to freely choose to smoke or not smoke. Both addiction and behaviour, and therefore interventions to change behaviour within public health, become issues of will and psychological cueing, which situate behaviour within the individual's head. Blame and responsibility also emerge from this understanding, as an ability to make 'health' choices is framed as an individual issue and cognitive decision.

However, such a framing misses the multiple interactions between people, e-cigarettes, places, other people and other objects, and the ways in which these may contribute to actions. Indeed, rather than being situated in the head, health practices can instead be seen to emerge from assemblages of elements—objects, people, places, etc. which act together. Through these understandings, e-cigarettes are not one thing, separate from space and time, but rather are objects that emerge relationally from particular circumstances, potentially shaping not only the relationships held with tobacco cigarettes, but also the varied relations which compose healthy, moral 'bodies' and indeed what addiction might mean and how this is experienced. Practices around e-cigarettes may configure new kinds of socio-material relations and lead us to ask new questions, not only about e-cigarettes but also about health, mind–body relationships and morality.

This understanding of people and objects as independent, bounded and disconnected from wider contexts, of course, means that RCTs generating a public health evidence base are better able to pin down the impact of objects. Conceptualising objects and people in this way makes them measurable and manageable, again situating responsibility within the individual. However, the material-semiotic practices of public health, through which debates and evidence-gathering on e-cigarette risk emerge, draw on particular fixed a priori assumptions to frame objects, people and the relationship between them—frames which not only miss but actively exclude alternative ways through which people might enact e-cigarettes. New practices, relationships and differing sociocultural patterns of smoking, some of the very aspects that researchers in this area declare they are interested in examining, may be found within the very relations that public health researchers have already presupposed. However, there are wider consequences of a shift to conceptualising objects as 'made' or enacted through practices. If e-cigarettes are constituted differently in different arenas and at different time periods, one fixed and definitive version of an e-cigarette cannot be captured in this way. How then might the riskiness of a technology be assessed? And if objects and individuals do not interact in such a manner, how might these affect conceptualisations of an individual responsibility for health?

Disagreements within the public health e-cigarette debate are unlikely to be resolved because both sides are in the end talking about different things. Different sides in the debate enact different objects through their practices and discourses, even if they draw on similar conceptualisations of objects, people and their relationship to do so. The e-cigarette-objects that emerge from each side may not be recognisable to e-cigarette smokers themselves. These practices and discourses set up their own socio-material relations. PMDs emerge from and impact on material-semiotic practices within medicine as well as outside it, no matter how static and separate medicine might frame these as being. Neither what an object 'is' nor whether it is 'risky' are therefore elements intrinsic to a particular technology, as technologies are not singular things. Instead, the qualities of objects are relational and emerge from how these are enacted in practices. 'Riskiness' emerges as an attribute ascribed by medicine as a future trajectory of just one of the multiple objects made through these different constructions.

Notes

1. It is debatable to what extent this 'denormalisation' has in reality occurred for all groups and across all spaces.
2. A growth and attention to risks in everyday life is also present in 'risk society' theorisations (e.g. Giddens, 1991; Beck, 1992) which suggest that while the past was previously drawn on to determine the present, the future- as constructed through various risk scenarios- is now used

to do so (Caplan, 2000). Late (or 'high') modernity has also promoted a scientific and rational worldview through which risk is framed and assessed (Giddens, 1991).

3. Coveney and Bunton's own work on drug taking seeks to address this lacuna, focusing specifically on the relationship between drug use and pleasure. It places pleasure within its wider social, cultural and historical context as an alternative approach to drug use in public health (Bunton & Coveney, 2011).

4. Bell and Keane (2012) point out that cigarette smoking does not fit with dominant models of addiction where addiction causes a person to behave badly- the smoker is able to live an ordinary and productive life and is not an 'out-of-control junkie governed by an unmanageable desire, at least until they try to quit' (2012, p.243). A notion of 'dependence' rather than 'addiction' has therefore often been attributed to cigarette use.

Acknowledgements Many thanks to Simon Cohn, Emma Garnett and Conor Farrington for their comments in the development of this chapter.

References

Abrams, D. B. (2014). Promise and peril of e-cigarettes: Can disruptive technology make cigarettes obsolete? *The Journal of the American Medical Association, 311*(2), 135–136.

ASH. (2016). Use of electronic cigarettes (vapourisers) among adults in Great Britain. Action on Smoking on Health (ASH) Fact sheet 33, April 2016. Available online at: http://www.ash.org.uk/files/documents/ASH_891.pdf. Accessed November 7, 2016.

Baudrillard, J. (1994/1981). *Simulcra and simulation*. Trans. S. F. Glaser. USA: University of Michigan Press.

Beck, U. (1992). *Risk society: Towards a new modernity*. London: Sage.

Bell, K., Salmon, A., Bowers, M., Bell, J., & McCullough, L. (2010). Smoking, stigma and tobacco 'denormalization': Further reflections on the use of stigma as a public health tool. A commentary on *Social Science and Medicine's* Stigma, prejudice, discrimination and health special issue (76: 3). *Social Science and Medicine, 70,* 795–799.

Bell, K., & Keane, H. (2012). Nicotine control: E-cigarettes, smoking and addiction. *International Journal of Drug Addiction, 23,* 242–247.

Benjamin, W. (1968/1955). The work of art in the age of mechanical reproduction. In H. Arendt (Ed.), *Illuminations* (pp. 214–218). London: Fontana.

Bennet, T. (2013). Habit: Time, freedom, governance. *Body & Society, 19*(2–3), 107–135.

Benson, P. (2010). Safe cigarettes. *Dialectical Anthropology, 34,* 49–56.

Britten, J., & Bogdanovica, I. (2014). *Electronic cigarettes. A report commissioned by Public Health England.* London: Health and Wellbeing Directorate, Public Health England. Available online at: https://www.gov.uk/government/uploads/system/uploads/attachment_data/file/311887/Ecigarettes_report.pdf. Accessed January 26, 2016.

Bunton, R., & Coveney, J. (2011). Drugs' pleasures. *Critical Public Health, 21,* 9–23.

Caplan, P. (2000). Introduction. In P. Caplan (Ed.), *Risk revisited* (pp. 1–28). London: Pluto Press.

Chapman, S. (2013). Should e-cigarettes be as freely available as tobacco? No. *British Medical Journal, 346,* 3840–3841.

Chapman, S. (2014). E-cigarettes: Does the new emperor of tobacco harm reduction have any clothes? *European Journal of Public Health, 24*(4), 535–536.

Conrad, P. (1992). Medicalization and Social Control. *Annual Review of Sociology, 18,* 209–232.

Cooper, A. J. M., Dearnley, K., Williams, K., et al. (2015). Protocol for the Get Moving trial: A randomised controlled trial to assess the effectiveness of minimal contact interventions to promote fitness and physical activity in an occupational health setting. *BMC Public Health, 15,* 296.

Coveney, J., & Bunton, R. (2003). In pursuit of the study of pleasure: Implications for health research and practice. *Health, 7,* 161–179.

De Andrade, M., Hastings, G., & Angus, K. (2013). Promotion of electronic cigarettes: Tobacco marketing reinvented? *British Medical Journal, 347,* 15–17.

Dew, K. (2012). *The cult and science of public health. A sociological investigation.* New York & Oxford: Berghahn Books.

Ecks, S. (2008). Three propositions for an evidence-based medical anthropology. *Journal of the Royal Anthropological Institute* (N.S.), S77–S92.

Etter, J. F. (2013). Should e-cigarettes be as freely available as tobacco? Yes. *British Medical Journal, 346,* 3845–3846.

Fairchild, A. L., Bayer, R., & Colgrove, J. (2014). The renormalization of smoking? E-cigarettes and the tobacco 'endgame'. *New England Journal of Medicine, 370,* 293–295.

Frazer, J. G. (1890). *The golden bough: A study in comparative religion.* London: Macmillan.

Giddens, A. (1991). *Modernity and self-identity: Self and society in the late modern age.* Cambridge: Polity Press.

Hajek, P. (2013). Electronic cigarettes for smoking cessation. *Lancet, 382,* 1614–1616.

Hsu, R., Myers, A. E., Ribisl, K. M., et al. (2013). An observational study of retail availability and in-store marketing of e-cigarettes in London: Potential to undermine recent tobacco control gains? *British Medical Journal Open, 3,* e004085.

Kandel, D. B. (2003). Does marijuana use cause the use of other drugs? *Journal of the American Medical Association, 289*(4), 482–483.

Klein, R. (1995). *Cigarettes are sublime.* Reading: Picador.

Law, J., & Singleton, V. (2005). Object lessons. *Organization, 12,* 331–355.

Lynch, R., & Cohn, S. (2015). In the loop: Practices of self-monitoring from accounts by trial participants. *Health: An Interdisciplinary Journal for the Social Study of Health Illness and Medicine, 20*(5), 523–538.

Maller, C. J. (2015). Understanding health through social practices: Performance and materiality in everyday life. *Sociology of Health & Illness, 37*(1), 52–66.

McKee, M., & Capewell, S. (2015). Electronic cigarettes: We need evidence, not opinions. *The Lancet, 386*(10000), 1239.

McNeill, A., Brose, L. S., Calder, R., Hitchman, S. C., Hajek, P., & McRobbie, H. (2015). *E-cigarettes: an evidence update. A report commissioned by Public Health England.* Crown Copyright.

Mol, A. (2002). *The body multiple: Ontology in medical practice.* Durham: Duke University Press.

Pols, J. (2012). *Care at a distance: On the closeness of technology.* Amsterdam: Amsterdam University Press.

The Publican's Morning Advertiser. (2013). 'Fuller's bans e-cigarettes from pubs' by Ellie Bothwell, 27th November 2013. Available online at: http://www.morningadvertiser.co.uk/Legal/Health-safety/Fuller-s-e-cigarettes. Accessed January 31, 2016.

Public Health England. (2015). E-cigarettes: A new foundation for evidence-based policy and practice. PHE publications gateway number: 2015260. Available online at: https://www.gov.uk/government/uploads/system/uploads/attachment_data/file/454517/Ecigarettes_a_firm_foundation_for_evidence_based_policy_and_practice.pdf. Accessed January 31, 2016.

Puhl, R. M., & Heuer, C. A. (2010). Obesity stigma: Important considerations for public health. *American Journal of Public Health, 100,* 1019–1028.

Stimson, G. V. (2014). Public health leadership and electronic cigarette users. *European Journal of Public Health, 24*(4), 534–535.

Taussig, M. (1993). *Mimesis and alterity: A particular history of the senses.* London: Routledge.

Part IV

Reconstructing the Device: Regulation, Commercialisation, and Design

Part IV of the book deepens our understanding of devices themselves by illustrating how PMDs can be considered as a nexus of issues of design, regulation, and capitalism in the context of emerging relationships between public and private sectors. Chapter 9 outlines the uncertain environment of existing and emerging regulatory regimes for medical devices before examining concrete processes of adoption through two case studies of PMDs that monitor blood flow and pressure. This chapter draws on the concept of 'technology identity' to emphasise how key features of specific devices shape the evaluative reactions of a range of stakeholders, with implications for potential use. Chapter 10 focuses on the entanglements between PMDs and contemporary capitalism, with particular attention to the use of PMDs in corporate wellness programmes. The resulting socio-technical assemblage allows companies to improve employees' health while simultaneously improving productivity, thus associating healthiness with 'activity' as a wider moral value. Chapter 11, lastly, considers PMDs as products of complex design processes that function as intersections of aesthetic and scientific agendas. Adopting a case study approach to the involvement of users in the co-design of orthotics, this chapter demonstrates how craft sensibilities can facilitate the creation of desirable PMDs, thus offering the potential to increase adherence over time. Throughout this Part of the book, PMDs are clearly shown as embedded within wider regulatory, economic, and material contexts which not only give sense to, but also derive new meanings from, individuals' health-focused interactions with new medical technologies in the form of PMDs.

9

Blood Informatics: Negotiating the Regulation and Usership of Personal Devices for Medical Care and Recreational Self-monitoring

Alex Faulkner

Introduction

Contemporary technological health care is characterised by a multitude of devices. Medical technologies are the product of global industries and the object of multidimensional marketing and regulation. Concepts of individual health and patienthood, and healthcare organisation and delivery, are being redefined by the emergence of personalising trends in disease risk profiling, diagnostics, health monitoring, telecare systems, individualised therapies, and personal mobile IT devices—though it is easy to overestimate and over-hype the significance of these trends. Trends of informaticisation, miniaturisation, digitalisation, molecularisation, geneticisation and cellularisation are all combining at the same moment in history. In everyday life, we thus increasingly inhabit

A. Faulkner (✉)
Centre for Global Health Policy, University of Sussex, Brighton, UK
e-mail: a.faulkner@sussex.ac.uk

© The Author(s) 2018   **203**
R. Lynch and C. Farrington (eds.), *Quantified Lives and Vital Data*,
Health, Technology and Society, https://doi.org/10.1057/978-1-349-95235-9_9

'a domain of highly technologized health care or 'techno-health', whether that be inside or outside formal healthcare systems.

Many, though not all, of the ubiquitous technologies of health care are 'medical devices'. The terminology of 'devices' invokes attention to the institutionalised medical device industries and sectors, and institutionalised medical device law, regulation and governance processes. Innovation of medical device technologies into society and the healthcare system is a process in which a variety of social, economic and medical interests and visions meet. The political economy of the European Union (EU) is important to the world of medical devices because of EU-wide regulatory regimes which define markets and the rules of engagement for trade in and with the European Economic Area. Social theory analysis points to the crucial part played by the definition of technical standards in the evolution of technological zones (Barry 2006; Faulkner 2009b) and political jurisdictions: the 'EU's governance blend… requires European domains to be constituted in order that they may be governed' (Delanty and Rumford 2005, p. 146). The extent and nature of standardisation achieved through specific regulatory regimes are crucial to an understanding of both the industrial economy and health protection through standards for the safety, quality and efficacy of devices entering the healthcare system. New technologies challenge 'inherited' regulatory regimes (Stokes 2012). The advent of mobile devices and downloadable software challenges conventional demarcations of the 'medical device industry' itself as a technological zone, the organisation of embedded 'healthcare systems' and the existing regulatory frameworks, as this chapter explores. As will be shown, gatekeepers in the form of both market access regulators and healthcare innovation institutions condition the trajectories and 'gateways' (Faulkner 2016) by which medical devices might be adopted in everyday practice.

Most germane to this chapter, digital devices, data and Internet communication are essential to an increasing proportion of these technologies. The current developments are starting to cross the boundaries of conventional medical care into the realms of lifestyle, culture and entertainment. The cultural appeal of gadgets has become an integral part of consumer cultures. The cultural and social appeal of such a 'euphoria of gadgets' was noted as long ago as the mid-twentieth century by

C.P. Snow (1961, reflecting on the UK government politics of technology during World War Two). C.P. Snow was a novelist and high-level civil servant, famous for the concept of 'the corridors of power' and the 'two cultures' thesis, though Snow cautioned that 'anyone who is drunk with gadgets is a menace'!

These developments are dovetailing with, and partly enabling, shifts in the medical paradigm for care of people living with and suffering from medical conditions, especially chronic illness, and policymakers and healthcare researchers are actively promoting technologies that might alleviate some of the burdens of care systems for people with such conditions who can live and act with some measure of autonomy. Thus, the gadgetry of mobile health (now conventionally abbreviated as 'mHealth') is being promoted in health policy too:

> mHealth technologies have the potential to change every aspect of the health care environment and to do so while delivering better outcomes and substantially lowering costs. For consumers, mHealth offers the promise of improved convenience, more active engagement in their care, and greater personalisation. For clinicians, mHealth could lead to reduced demands on their time and permit them to instead refocus on the art of medicine. Much remains to be done to drive this transformation. Most critically needed is real-world clinical trial evidence to provide a roadmap for implementation that confirms its benefits to consumers, clinicians, and payers alike. (Steinhubl et al. 2013)

In this context, the chapter is divided into two parts, the first locating the emergence of personal medical devices in the context of governance, risk management and regulatory regime-building, and the second part analysing actual and potential usership processes of adoption and 'domestication' of devices both within and outside organised healthcare delivery systems, the UK's National Health Service being the main reference point. To clarify the aim of this chapter further, although there are important aspects of mHealth innovation that concern personal and social identity, patienthood, embodiment and dependence/autonomy, these are not the focus here. The discussion is on the structural gatekeeping processes and epistemic semiotics shaping personal and systemic mHealth device innovation, rather than on the 'lived experience' or health-related phenomenology of their use (such as discussed by Lupton 2013, 2014a, b).

In order to contrast different types and configurations of 'personal' device, I focus on case studies of devices associated with medical conditions, therapies and health risks connected to the working of the vascular system, that is, the circulation of blood in the human body. Blood can be the carrier of disease, may itself be diseased or under-performing and may be used diagnostically as an indicator of a range of medical conditions and to monitor health and disease states. The devices I use to inform the discussion therefore are, first, the coagulometer, used for self-monitoring of anticoagulation treatment for a variety of circulatory conditions and risks; second, the blood pressure (BP) monitor, especially smartphone-based applications (apps). These two cases can be taken as representing two extremes of self-monitoring devices: the smartphone app technology being a consumer product, ultra-mobile, one application amongst many on the smartphone platform, usable outside formal medical healthcare systems, and the coagulometer highly medicalised, strongly embedded in healthcare systems and medical expertise, less transportable and dedicated to a single function. Before embarking on these case studies of innovation and usership, this section of this chapter deals with the framing of mHealth/personal medical devices, and especially their framing within legal, regulatory frameworks. Because the UK's regulation for medical devices and pharmaceuticals responds to the European Union (EU) legislation and debate, the EU level is the primary focus. It has to be noted that the UK population voted by a majority to leave the EU in the referendum of June 2016 ('Brexit'). While there will doubtless be changes to the relevant regulatory frameworks following from this, and details are yet to be worked out let alone implemented at the time of writing, it is likely that the emerging UK-based regulatory regimes will remain at least in principle equivalent to those currently in force or under development. Therefore, this chapter continues to present the currently prevailing EU regulatory regimes in the likelihood that the issues and broadly defined regulatory domains will not change markedly in the near future.

Framing and Regulating Mobile Medical Devices

The aim of this section is to show how politico-economic regimes of standards and regulations with different classes of risk and data requirements for placing devices on the market, applicable in the European Union, shape the innovation context for technology developers and distributors; and also to show how the emergence of devices with a citizen/patient user interface is being framed and regulated, thus defining the types of claims producers can legitimately make about the appropriate use of their devices. Notably, to anticipate this section of this chapter, such regulations attempt to define the boundary between medical and non-medical use, and to protect individual data privacy. The scope of medical devices globally is vast, and significant as an economic sector. Estimates in the region of 10,000 device families and 400,000 different devices are not uncommon. Safety standards are supported by European directives for devices that provide a definite medical intervention.

The framing of new technological zones is achieved in large part through the legal force of regulatory frameworks. It is clear that in approaching the emergence of personal medical or health technologies, a range of alternative framings have been coined and variously supported in the field, each with different connotations and implications. The significance of the 'mHealth' and 'eHealth' categories should be considered in the light of pre-existing, inherited regulatory categories. The primary context of existing regulation for personal mobile medical or health devices is the EU's Medical Device Directives, established during the 1990s and being revised in order to strengthen them in the mid-2010s, with a new, somewhat more stringent Medical Device Regulation coming into force in 2017. The European Commission has published established guidance on the classification of medical devices. The risk-related philosophy underlying this is:

> … a classification concept which is essentially based on potential hazards related to the use and possible failure of devices taking account of technology used and of health policy considerations. This approach in turn allows the use of a small set of criteria that can be combined in various

ways: duration of contact with the body, degree of invasiveness and local vs. systemic effect. (EC DG Enterprise 2001, p. 3)

A medical device is defined as 'any instrument, apparatus, appliance, software, material or other article, whether used alone or in combination, including the software intended by its manufacturer to be used specifically for diagnostic and/or therapeutic purposes and necessary for its proper application'. The corporeal starting point of the above definition results in groupings, not mutually exclusive, that include: devices with a measuring function; active devices; implantable devices; and invasive devices. 'Active implantable' devices and 'devices for in vitro diagnosis' are separate groups again, and in Europe are covered by separate legislative acts. All software that meets the definition, including software that works in combination with a physical device, for instance a smartphone, will meet the criteria of medical device. Clearly, in the case of mHealth devices, the regulatory framings of devices with a measuring function and possibly in vitro diagnosis will apply. However, it is also obvious that the 'regulatory connection' (Brownsword 2008) between medical device categories and mHealth/personal device innovations is far from close, mainly due to the informatics and data processing aspects of the latter. Thus, given the yawning gap in regulatory connection between the new mHealth technologies and inherited medical device regulatory regimes, it is necessary to investigate how the EU is responding to the personal mobile medicine and mobile health challenge.

In spite of the strong claims of the existing medical device regime, in a striking framing move, mHealth technologies have in fact become also framed as part of the European Commission's 'Digital Agenda for Europe'. In 2014, the European Commission published a Green Paper on mobile health with a public consultation, in which it invited stakeholders to provide their views on eleven identified barriers to the uptake of mHealth in the EU (European Commission 2015a). These included 'access of web entrepreneurs to the mHealth market'. In this framing, mHealth is seen as part of 'eHealth', and notably includes applications which: 'perform measurements (e.g. of glucose levels); complement medical devices (e.g. helping in the delivery of insulin by transmitting control signals to the pump …); remind patients they should take their medication; provide recommendations … to improve users' overall health & wellbeing' (European Commission 2015b). Here, mHealth is defined as: 'medical and public health practice supported by mobile devices, such as mobile phones, patient monitoring devices, personal digital assistants (PDAs), and other wireless devices' (World Health Organisation 2014; cited in Green Paper 2014). mHealth 'also includes applications … such as lifestyle and wellbeing apps that may connect to medical devices or sensors (e.g. bracelets or watches) as well as personal guidance systems, health information and medication reminders provided by sms and telemedicine provided wirelessly' (Green Paper, p. 3).

Thus, we see in this extraordinarily wide-ranging definition a joining-together of medical device categories such as monitoring and sensing devices, with new categories such as 'personal digital assistants'. Given that many mHealth devices will incorporate medical programs, software and communications, the medical device Directives are extremely important to their regulation, but the 'digital society' definition also encompasses non-medical functions of consumer products with various possible 'health' applications. The importance of this distinction is illustrated in the discussion of the blood-monitoring devices below. The Medical Device Directives have been under debate and revision during the 2010s, largely in the wake of safety scandals. However, the proposed revision has been criticised as not explicitly tackling the mHealth apps issues: 'The premise that such apps are of "low risk" seems to be dubious, especially given the increasing use of such apps by both patients and physicians in medical treatment and diagnosis' (Quinn et al. 2013, p. 202). Thus, there remains a notable unresolved ambiguity in the applicability of the two regulatory regimes, the devices regime established, though of questionable stringency and lagging behind in the mHealth arena, and the 'digital society' regime emerging.

It is impossible to discuss the regulation of mHealth without touching on issues of data privacy. The key EU regulation is Directive *95/46/EC* on the protection of individuals with regard to the processing of personal data and on the free movement of such data, commonly known as the 'Data Protection Directive' (Quinn et al. 2013), in which data protection is recognised and protected as a fundamental right.

In a forthcoming General Data Protection Regulation (GDPR), expected for approval in 2016, the European Commission intends to strengthen data protection for individuals and regulate export of personal data outside the EU, of obvious importance for Internet-connected technologies. The Commission's primary objectives of GPRS are to 'give citizens back the control of their personal data and to simplify the regulatory environment for international business by unifying the regulation within the EU'. The Data Protection Directive allows for processing of medical data where 'explicit consent' is obtained.

Legal analysis of the applicability of data protection laws (in Europe) has surmised that 'mHealth services may therefore be faced with the need to seek consent on a much more regular basis than is needed for conventional medical services'. New mechanisms might be needed to make consent for data transfer possible: 'These include the possibility to appoint a third party for consent, perhaps a specialist agency tasked with dealing with such issues for many patients' (Quinn et al. 2013, pp. 203–204). It may also be possible to adapt the concept of a 'healthcare institution' so that it would include 'virtual institutions that may be connected through their practice if not through their geographic proximity' (Quinn et al. 2013, pp. 203–204). However, it can be very difficult to assess whether mHealth apps collect 'sensitive' data. Thus, data protection issues enter into the borderline between medical devices and applications targeting non-medical health status monitoring. In this light, it is useful to contrast the respective responses to the European Commission Green Paper, from EUCOMED, the EU level medical device trade association, and EPHA, the European Public Health Alliance.

EUCOMED's formal response to the Green Paper consultation includes:

> 1. Software packages and Apps which collect and store data which is pertinent to the private usage of an individual could be presented within a medical category but with a specific filter or listing, clearly defining them as fully regulated "Medical Devices" or as "Health and Well-Being" Apps. 2. All "Medical Devices" software should require that the device

is "locked down" with a minimum level of security via finger-print or a numeric access code. (EUCOMED 2014)

EPHA's (European Public Health Alliance) response includes:

[T]he Green Paper states that 9 out of 20 health-related apps have been found to transmit data to private companies tracking mobile phone use. This is clearly not acceptable and there needs to be a clear distinction between health - which is a personal right and also benefits society as a whole – and consumer goods bought and sold for profit-making purposes. Moreover, pharmaceutical companies themselves may be behind apps without this necessarily being obvious to the user. (EPHA 2014)

It is clear that ambiguity in the important use of terms to denote the emerging fields is apparent in these statements; EUCOMED distinguishing between 'medical' and 'health and wellbeing', while EPHA distinguishes between 'health' devices (apparently close to EUCOMED's 'medical device') and consumer products. These differing framings highlight that there is an interest-based politics of categorisations which are important to defining the safety and human rights environments in which borderlines between medical and 'nonmedical' devices are being drawn.

In summary, regulation shapes the context in which manufacturers and developers may design and claim intended use of their products, and personal devices with medical and health-related applications are currently subject to a politics of regulatory negotiation. The emergence of self-monitoring devices is of great concern to regulators, both in medicine and in business. The regulatory frameworks are evolving and overlapping, and currently are not well adapted to self-monitoring technology—a clear case of 'regulatory lag'. The conflict and ambiguity between medical device-based safety regulation and the 'digital society' ambition is acute. Public health perspectives are suspicious of commercial developers entering the marketplace from a non-medical base.

Given this important but complex and uncertain regulatory environment, I now turn to consider the multiple factors shaping the adoption of self-monitoring devices in two case studies of blood-monitoring technologies, in which innovators must respond to, and to some extent anticipate, this evolving environment. As this discussion will show, regulation of the claims that producers can make is just one of the dynamics shaping the market context in which personal medical or health devices may be adopted in practice. Leaving aside direct insight into users' motivations and socio-economic situations, which are not dealt with here, the role of consumer marketing, the mass media commentary, clinical opinion about scientific evidence, technology interfaces, public health and healthcare policy, and formal health technology assessment institutions also all play a part in the contrasting exemplar cases below.

Adoption and Usership

Turning to uptake of devices by users, the concept of 'technology identity' (Ulucanlar et al. 2013) is used here to discuss the way in which users (citizens, patients, health professionals, healthcare planners and purchasers) understand, evaluate, and actually or potentially acquire and use such technologies. This concept aims to bridge between the concepts of technological determinism and the social determinism of constructivist theory (Timmermans and Berg 2003). Technology identities are theorised as being forged and typically contested in a sociotechnical 'adoption space' which is negotiated between stakeholders around given technologies. The concept draws on actor-network theory and technology 'affordances' (Hutchby 2001), which are seen as endowing technology itself with an active status in the production and direction of sociotechnical innovation. The notion of affordances has been used in other conceptualisations of mHealth innovation and its social significance: 'The technical affordances (of apps) structure the ways in which they are used and the meanings that are ascribed to them' (Lupton 2014c; my parentheses). Here, the adoption space includes the mass media, 'evidence' debates, marketing, IT capabilities and policymakers, as well as regulation.

Technology identity is defined as: 'A narrative or discursive presence of the technology that delineates a particular set of attributed characteristics and performative expectancies as representative of the technology's distinctiveness and value' (Ulucanlar et al. 2013). Identities are collaboratively constructed through claim-making and counter-claim-making: 'stories, both enthusiastic and sceptical, are exchanged at a variety of interactional spaces' (ibid). The concept also resonates with kindred concepts in the sociology of technology, such as that of 'domestication' (Silverstone and Haddon 1996). Five primary dimensions of technology identity have been derived from medical device case studies (Ulucanlar et al. 2013): Biography, Effectiveness, Utility, Risk and Requirements, the latter referring to the constrained affordances which technologies may enact. Without rehearsing here the details of these five dimensions, the following accounts note key features of two case studies of blood and pressure monitoring devices, relating them to the five identity domains.

As noted above, this chapter takes as its case studies two types of device that use blood and blood flow as metric materials for the monitoring of medical conditions. One is typically used by self-monitoring patients as part of clinical regimes in interaction with healthcare professionals, while the other may typically be used with little or no oversight by medical professionals. However, both are used for monitoring high-risk medical conditions and associated drug therapies, which can lead to severe and life-threatening events. In conceptual terms, both are highly flexible, 'configurational' technologies (Fleck 1994), which afford multiple possible modes and styles of usership. As mentioned in the Introduction, the two cases are the coagulometer, used for self-monitoring of anticoagulation treatment for certain circulatory conditions and risks, and the blood pressure (BP) monitor, especially smartphone-based applications. I discuss each of these in terms of their actual and potential technology identity in their multidimensional adoption spaces below. In the case of the coagulometer, I draw on a UK research project that investigated the processes of adoption or non-adoption of various devices in the NHS (Tomlin et al. 2013); in the case of the BP monitor, I draw on a range of public information sources, primarily academic journal articles and website sources.

The Thickness of Blood: Risky Responsibilities

Coagulometers are used for measuring and monitoring the viscosity of blood in the case of drug therapy for a variety of heart and circulatory conditions that might produce potentially dangerous blood clotting. It is estimated that some 950,000 people currently use long-term oral anti-coagulation therapy (OAT) in the UK. Chronic medical conditions for which blood-thinning drugs (mainly warfarin in the UK) may be administered include heart disease, deep vein thrombosis (DVT), stroke or stroke risk and patients with artificial heart valves. There is a strong, organised patient advocacy movement to promote the direct use of this device by patients. Most patient-users of the device monitor their blood coagulation, but some also manage their own drug dosage. Although the potential use of the device is in the hundreds of thousands in the UK, actual use is quite low, estimated at around 25–30,000 at the time of writing. Some public healthcare regimes such as Germany have actively introduced home monitoring technologies, including the full cost of reimbursement, but other countries including the UK have been less enthusiastic. Versions of the device are produced by several device manufacturers, by far the largest of which globally is Roche Diagnostics.

The development of portable, handheld versions of the device has occurred only over the last 25 years, and thus this technology appears in a context in which specialised health professional expertise and organisation are already institutionalised. The traditional service model for managing such patients has been periodic visits to consultant haematology clinics and interpretation of tests in pathology laboratories, a lengthy process. To characterise the technology itself, the self-monitoring device comprises a unit slightly larger and heavier than a mobile/cell phone, with a small screen that provides a digital display; it also includes small test strips containing a reagent, lancets for obtaining fingertip blood and a quality control liquid solution. Users have to obtain a trace of blood and place it on the strip, which is then inserted in the device. Systems produce the 'INR' (International Normalised Ratio) digital numeric indicator as a readout on the display screen, indicating how fluid or viscous the blood flow is, and this has to be kept strictly within a narrow 'therapeutic range'. These affordances of the technology clearly *require* a range of abilities on the part of the user, and medical knowledge and facilities.

Turning to the coagulometer's informatics, the INR ratio normally has to be communicated to a clinic(ian) to consider if the drug dosage needs to be altered. Self-monitoring patients will typically be expected by medical professionals to remain connected to some extent to regimes of care in a clinic-based system in order to record and communicate INR readings. Traditionally, the readings are recorded in a booklet given to the patient. With a self-monitoring system, this is usually done now by the patient via low-tech electronic communication, e.g. email or telephone. Here again, the device's affordances allow a high degree of mobility in the part of users, provided that the device is at hand when necessary.

Policy in the UK in this field has been piecemeal and local practices vary widely. The devices are not funded currently via the UK NHS. Patient advocacy groups such as the British Cardiac Patients Association and Anticoagulation Europe are prominent in promoting self-monitoring, linking with manufacturers and clinician-champions, raising funds for coagulometers, being represented on Department of Health policy groups and negotiating on policy issues, such as the NHS prescription status for testing strips. A small number of hospital-based clinical centres are known to support local initiatives, but these are uncoordinated (Faulkner 2009a). This is a field where industry and voluntary organisations are powerful drivers, having some limited success in influencing healthcare policy, campaigns raising the distinctiveness of the technology, part of its biographical identity, in the eyes of policymakers embracing empowerment agendas.

The regulatory status and applicable standards are important to shaping the identity of the coagulometer. Coagulometer manufacturers are regulated within the EU as diagnostic medical devices under the In Vitro Diagnostic Device Directive. They must, therefore, have been certified for safety and the Directive requires that devices for self-testing must take into account the likely level of skill of the intended user and the influence on the test result that could come from variation in technique and environment. Instructions for use should state that decisions about medical treatment should not be taken without consultation with a medical practitioner. There is, therefore, a variety of legislative and less formal regulation affecting coagulometer adoption. In the UK, it is clear that assessment of safety requires consideration of the usership context in which the device is employed. In terms of this device's technology identity, we can see that the 'risk identity' is very much dependent on the perspectives of stakeholders on users' ability to use the device correctly as a 'technology-in-practice', rather than its technical safety as a machine.

The device's 'effectiveness identity' has been greatly contested over the last 15–20 years. There has been a divergence of opinion about the evidence of effectiveness of self-monitoring amongst clinicians, and a divergence of medical specialists' attitudes towards experimental schemes to introduce self-monitoring. Specialist medical professions, especially those in haematology, are reluctant to cede control over their conventional expertise. In the community, GPs also found it difficult to relinquish control over the monitoring function (Tomlin et al. 2013). The nervousness around self-monitoring was compounded by the conviction that the GP remained 'vaguely responsible' for potential adverse events. Nevertheless, many studies internationally suggest that patient self-monitoring has equivalent or better control of INR levels. A number of recent wide-ranging systematic reviews using secondary analysis have quite recently appeared. One such systematic review and meta-analysis conducted under the auspices of the high-status Cochrane Collaboration and published in *The Lancet* consolidates the view that self-testing was at least as effective clinically as standard methods (Heneghan et al. 2006).

Tomlin et al.'s study found that GPs did not offer self-monitoring routinely, limiting it to those who asked for it and were deemed capable (such as younger people, professionals, university professors, haematologists), thus constructing a strong resistive identity around perceived risk. Thus, this research showed that amongst clinicians there was at least an imputed 'utility identity' that may well have been leading to systematic reluctance to offer the technology as an option to large groups of potential users, or to commission it as part of anticoagulation services (Tomlin et al. 2013).

In the case of the UK, the technology, apart from the prescribable testing strips, has the marketplace status of a consumer product. It may be that although this clearly limits the socio-economic range from which the majority of users are likely to come, and thus inequities in access are likely to remain, there may be some psychological reward and contribution to motivation and self-concept that this structural circumstance promotes. In summary, the configuring of coagulometer users may be as much due to the socio-economic circumstance of the diffusion routes of the device as to the qualities of the device itself, the care milieu and professional opinion.

The coagulometer's future was seen as uncertain at the beginning of the 2010s, but since then the main provider of the technology has been successful in achieving a (non-mandatory) recommendation by NICE for selected patients:

> The NICE diagnostics guidance on self-monitoring coagulometers supports the use of the Coaguchek XS system (Roche Diagnostics) and the InRatio2 PT/INR Monitor (Alere) as options for some adults with atrial fibrillation or heart valve disease who are on long-term anticoagulation therapy…. to self-monitor…Because self-monitoring provides almost instant results, self-monitoring can reduce anxiety, provide a sense of control for the patient and remove the need to frequently attend clinics or hospitals. (NICE 2014)

And:

> The NICE Health Technologies Adoption Programme is currently working with a number of NHS organisations to produce an adoption support resource for self-monitoring coagulation status… (NICE 2014)

In summary, as with all testing devices, accuracy and safety depended on the user's expertise and system-wide safeguards such as accreditation, internal and external quality control procedures and regular auditing. These socio-clinical norms about risk and control have impacted on the adoptability of the coagulometer and the size of its market. Having diffused relatively little during many years when it benefited from an insecure clinical rationale, it appears that the recent intervention of NICE in the UK will lead to increasing acceptance of the technology-in-practice amongst clinicians broadly. Interestingly, NICE's support-ive decision has brought 'user confidence' to the fore in the discursive identity of this device. However, the consumer status of the device as a personal expense will obviously remain an impediment to widespread use, though NICE's decision will likely lead to increased pressure on service commissioners for funding for selected patients as part of anti-coagulation services. Such developments will still require resolution of ambivalence and ambiguity around clinical protocols to define lines of responsibility. In general, however, there is a paucity of research on the everyday experience of communication media and information flows with coagulometers, regardless of the care setting.

Blood Pressures: Measuring, Estimating or Monitoring?

The aim of this section is to present a comparison with the coagulom-eter case by examining the emerging epistemic space of mobile blood pressure(BP) device innovations. This section draws largely on pub-lished sources of various kinds, including companies' marketing mate-rial and websites, medical and scientific commentary and research, users' online comments on particular apps, device and app user guides, and regulator reports. While BP is measured in most healthcare sites by a medicalised device combining digital technology with a pressuris-ing cuff, the appearance of smartphone-based applications claimed to monitor or in some cases measure BP is relatively new. As noted in the introduction, by focusing here on the smartphone app technology, I am examining a case at the opposite end of the spectrum from the highly medicalised, health system-embedded coagulometer. Blood pressure is an indicator of high-risk medical conditions, and its measurement has become involved in telematics innovations, for example:

> One of every 3 adults in the United States has hypertension…Despite this… less than half of individuals with hypertension have their blood pressure under control. A new generation of blood pressure cuffs for

home use can wirelessly transmit individual readings or long-term trends to a clinician, allowing for rapid feedback. (Steinhubl et al. 2013)

A huge variety of devices have been created, with different designs, with and without the pressurising cuff, with a variety of possible medical institutional arrangements for patients, or none at all. Names such as '*Blood Pressure Companion*'; and '*BP Watch*' are proliferating.

Locating BP apps in the context of all medical smartphone apps, it can be noted that 'mobile users disproportionally favored *tracking* tools' (Chang et al. 2011, my emphasis); Lupton has noted that 'working out' dominates the top ten Apple pay-for medical apps, although one of these is for high BP ("Blood Pressure Diary"). This app involves users 'uploading their bodily data to the app' (Lupton 2014c). Thus, many of the applications are essentially data recording systems that can analyse and present data once they have been obtained by other methods, for example producing graphs of BP trend over time. Nevertheless, there are a number of apps available for which producers do claim to measure, or in most producers' terminology 'estimate' BP:

> Researchers analysed the top 107 apps for 'hypertension' and 'high blood pressure' that are available for download on the Google Play store and Apple iTunes and found that nearly three-quarters offered tools for tracking medical data. But they also found seven Android apps that claimed users needed only to press their fingers onto phone screens or cameras to get blood-pressure readings – claims that scientists say are bogus. (*Daily Mail*, 26 December, 2014)

For example, the 'Instant Blood Pressure' app 'lets you measure your BP using only your (i)Phone – no cuff required' (www.instantbloodpressure.com). This app uses 'a patent-pending process developed by a team of forward-thinking biomedical engineers and software developers at AuraLife, a California-based digital health startup on 'a mission to help people better access health insight'. The company website states that '[u]sing only your smartphone and our proprietary algorithm, our app is intended to estimate your blood pressure before, during, and after recreational activities'. Its operation is simple: 'Place Finger Over Rear

Camera Lens/Press Phone Into Your Chest Over Your Heart (Finger still in place)/Quietly Hold Position for < 35 s And See Results'. A red warning at the top of the homepage states: 'Do not rely on *Instant Blood Pressure* for medical advice or diagnosis. It is not a replacement or substitute for a cuff or other blood pressure monitor' (company website).

Giving a sense of the public domains in which discourse about such devices circulates, high-profile technology magazine *Wired* has produced a feature on these BP applications. Noting an editorial in the *New England Journal of Medicine*, it refers to an Associate Professor of law in Dallas, Texas, who 'called attention to this problem', adding that 'you'll hear much the same complaint from (name) a medical doctor and director of the Scripps Translational Science Institute'. The article continues:

> These apps have no validated data compared with accepted reference standards and therefore are quite concerning …There is no public research explaining how the app operates, and the company hasn't done the kind of study that the Food and Drug Administration would require in order to get Instant Blood Pressure cleared as a medical device … the 'company's warning that the software is for recreational use only. (McMillan 2014)

The way in which the regulatory environment and clinical opinion and its representation in popular media impact on the app innovation process is evident in the above. Corporate giants of the computer, smartphone and communications gadget world are currently developing suites of health-related applications. For example, Apple's 'Health' app marketing (in January 2015 associated with UK's largest communications company BT) claims: 'The ability to test blood pressure and monitor heart conditions right from an iPhone could be a life-saver' (Hattersley 2015). Measuring BP is claimed to be one of the 'most requested' features, and there is already a device called the *QardioArm* that measures your BP and heart rate. The QardioArm looks like a regular arm cuff that a nurse would use, but is attached to a white box that transmits the information to the iPhone. The user wraps the QardioArm around their arm and presses the *Start* button on the iPhone app; it then tightens up and measures their blood pressure. A graph indicates whether users' BP is in the normal or hypertension range, and it can also detect irregular heartbeat activity. The web page states that '[h]aving access to the data about yourself is going to make a big difference when you visit a doctor' (cited in Hattersley 2015). Online comments from anonymous readers of this web page were sceptical either about the technology or about its potential users:

King Bertie	What a joke! …it can't even make a successful telephone call.
Wendylou68	Sound's ideal for a hypochondriac.

Data security issues were mentioned above in the section on regulation. Although it is difficult without empirical research (and possibly even with it) to assess the data-sharing aspects of these types of apps, some indication can be derived from the secondary sources used here. Legal commentary suggests that lack of regulatory clarity is leading Apple to be cautious about developing this suite of applications, especially regarding legal rules about privacy (Kelly 2014). In another example, the 'BP Watch' (not a timepiece) app on Android 'will help you record, track, analyse and share your blood pressure everywhere you go' (company website). The app offers various data-sharing facilities including 'Email, Skype, and Wifi Direct'. The user guide states that 'You can create profiles for each of your family members or friends'; creating a 'BP Watch account' requires the provision of personal data including name, age and gender (user guide http://numbersmatter2.me/?page_id=31).

The example highlights that in the case of BP measurement, there is a clear need for the interface with medical IT systems, where sought by patient or medical professional, to exist and to be compatible. Recent evaluation shows that this is a very challenging practical issue:

the inability of most electronic medical record systems to receive and process information from mobile devices continues to be a major impediment in realising the full potential of mHealth technology. (Logan 2013)

Blood pressure monitoring is a site of major continuing technological innovation and a diversifying range of devices, software applications and models of the communication interface. In the emerging usership of these devices, vexatious issues of personal identity and technology identity are becoming interlinked around digital personal data and their various platform technologies. From a medical point of view, IT-facilitated healthcare systems may benefit public health:

> Studies from our group in hypertension and other chronic conditions have shown improved health outcomes using mHealth applications that have undergone rigourous (*sic*) usability testing. (Logan et al. 2007)

In order to understand the above formulations of BP monitoring devices, I return to the notion of technology identity. What aspects of technology identity are being formed in these promissory and evaluative discourses? How is the 'adoption space' (Ulucanlar et al. 2013; Tomlin et al. 2013) of BP self-monitoring being shaped? Fox (2015) has usefully proposed that the 'relations' of the standard BP monitor are 'assembled' by at least these actors: 'vascular system—device—user—manufacturer—biomedicine – health professionals' (to which list we might add: regulators and healthcare researchers—who may be health professionals).

The discourses and evaluative commentary presented above enable us to interpretively characterise the emergent adoption space of BP smartphone apps to some extent. Key dimensions of the BP app adoption space are therefore: a global marketplace; data connectivity; data and their organisation; functionality; portability; regulatory uncertainty; and the healthcare/health professional interface. Most obviously, in terms of technology identity, the sociotechnical 'utility' of these gadgets appears the subject of disparate identity claims between manufacturers and health professionals, with BP *measuring* being especially contentious, and challenging the regulatory definitions outlined above. Although producers' claims might include non-liability notices and description of the device's function as 'estimates', whether potential and actual users will perceive the data produced by the device in this way in domestic and mobile environments remains a matter for empirical investigation. The use of the term 'estimate' or 'recreational' enables device and software app developers to remain legally outside the bounds of the medical device regulations, though contentiously so. The online availability of the apps means users are configured as private consumers rather than medical patients, an affordance of the technological set-up and marketplace. Further 'utility' may be afforded by the cultural appeal of smartphone technology seen to be 'cool' and offering access to Quantified Self communities (see Dudhwala, this volume). The *requirement* for healthcare system data- receiving infrastructure represents an impediment for medicalising use of the technology. Health professionals such as cardiologists may perceive a threat to technical standards in BP measurement. For businesses, an ambiguous identity of medical function device versus lifestyle gadget may be seen as an obstacle. Data privacy is a major concern with mHealth/apps in general. Lupton (2014c) cites a market research report of a survey of more than 2000 health and medical app developers, reporting 'that data security and standards issues were viewed as barriers to further development of this app market' (Jahns 2014).

Conclusion: The Boundary of Personal Medicine and Recreational Health

The authority and social legitimacy of institutional biomedicine and clinic-centred healthcare systems remain powerful while being challenged by the cases discussed above. Comparing these cases to other informatics-enabled healthcare innovations, we can note that the introduction into healthcare systems of telemedicine technologies was far less extensive than many early commentators predicted (May et al. 2003), and the same may be the case for the potentially even more individualised mHealth medical technologies. Likewise, medical regulators, although chasing fast-moving technology developments, are making efforts to defend the safety of people using technologies and software *as* medical devices. However, as shown in the section above on regulation, conflicting regulatory regimes and conflicting interests are currently confusing this effort. This chapter emphasises how, and to what extent, these technologies challenge both regulatory boundaries and standards, and the boundaries shaping the interactions of citizens and patients with organised, professional healthcare systems. In the process, the boundaries between the lifestyle-oriented device and the health system-embedded device are thrown into relief. The fact of app developers marketing products for 'recreational' use highlights the issue of a contested political discourse over medical versus lifestyle or well-being definitions, underpinned by regulatory borderlines, and use of these technologies. While the direction of European regulation of the mHealth field is geared to developing the field and facilitating the enterprise of app developers, neither the healthcare infrastructure nor health professional opinion currently supports apps which claim a BP measuring function, even if couched with small print eschewing medical responsibility. In this case, available technology potentially poses a risk to health—a risk that requires research to assess.

The 'technology identity' of the devices discussed here embody a stark contrast, with the coagulometer being relatively clear in its medical function and setting while the smartphone BP app shows significant ambiguity. The two case studies highlight the importance of the communication interface between citizens or patients and health professionals and a healthcare system, and the extent and technological means by which such communication is mediated if undertaken by remote, non-face-to-face methods. Research should explore what developers' 'recreational' framing means for users and their interaction with medical systems. It is known that patients can develop extremely detailed personal understandings of their own medical and personal device use; this is not simply 'recreational' or a leisure activity but rather amounts to a form of personal labour. The degree to which such self-labour might be authentically self-directed, autonomous and 'personal' as opposed to medically connected and supervised, is highlighted by the two case studies. From a public health point of view, there is a risk that use of certain devices may be *more* personal—isolated from medical practitioners and others and thus *too personal*—than envisioned by developers and other promoters of the technology.

Finally, the issues of data protection and consent to data sharing with device producers or distributors, and with healthcare providers, will become increasingly important as part of the identity of Internet and communications-enabled self-monitoring technologies.

Personal data sharing in online forums is enabled by some of these devices, as in the growing Quantified Self movement. Large scale future mobile technology-enabled self-monitoring would require re-design of both medical institutions, and raises the possibility, as Quinn et al. (2013) noted, that society may require the building of new virtual institutions to deal with the processing of high volume streams of personal, appropriately consented, vital data.

Acknowledgements A version of parts of this chapter was presented at the Wellcome Trust/University of Cambridge Symposium 'Theorising Personal Medical Devices: New Perspectives', Cambridge, UK, 18–19 September 2014. I am grateful for comments from participants.

References

Barry, A. (2006). Technological zones. *European Journal of Social Theory, 9*(2), 239–253.

Brownsword, R. (2008). So what does the world need now: Reflections on regulating technologies. In R. Brownsword & K. Yeung (Eds.), *Regulating technologies: Legal futures, regulatory frames, and technological fixes* (pp. 23–48). Portland: Hart Publishing.

Chang, L., Qing, Z., Holroyd, K., & Seng, E. (2011). Status and trends of mobile-health applications for iOS devices: A developer's perspective. *Journal of Systems and Software, 84*(11), 2022–2033.

Delanty, D., & Rumford, C. (2005). *Rethinking Europe: Social theory and the implications of Europeanization.* London: Routledge.

EC DG Enterprise. (2001). *Guidelines for the classification of medical devices.* Brussels: European Commission.

EPHA. (2014). (Response to) *Public consultation on the Commission's Green Paper on mobile health.* Available online at: 4-contributionsfromorganisationsDtoE.pdf. Accessed December 2015.

EUCOMED. (2014). (Response to) *Public consultation on the Commission's Green Paper on mobile health.* Available online at: 4-contributionsfromorganisationsDtoE.pdf. Accessed December 2015.

European Commission. (2015a). *Public consultation on the Green Paper on mobile Health.* Available online at: https://ec.europa.eu/digital-agenda/en/public-consultation-green-paper-mobile-health. Accessed January 2016.

European Commission. (2015b). *mHealth in Europe: Preparing the ground – consultation results published*. Available online at https://ec.europa.eu/digital-agenda/en/news/mhealth-europe-preparing-ground-consultation-results-published-today. Accessed January 2016.

Faulkner, A. (2009a). *Medical technology into healthcare and society: A sociology of devices, innovation and governance*. Basingstoke: Palgrave Macmillan.

Faulkner, A. (2009b). Regulatory policy as innovation: Constructing rules of engagement of a technological zone for tissue engineering in the European Union. *Research Policy, 38*(4), 637–646.

Faulkner, A. (2016). Opening the gateways to market and adoption of regenerative medicine? The UK case in context. *Regenerative Medicine, 11*(3), 321–330.

Fleck, J. (1994). Learning by trying—The implementation of configurational technology. *Research Policy, 23*(6), 637–652.

Fox, N. (2015). Personal health technologies, micropolitics and resistance: A new materialist analysis. *Health*. Online: http://hea.sagepub.com/content/early/2015/07/24/1363459315590248.

Hattersley, L. (2015). How your iPhone can monitor your health. Available online at: http://home.bt.com/tech-gadgets/phones-tablets/how-your-iphone-can-monitor-your-health-11363934390111. Accessed January 2016.

Heneghan, C., Alonso-Coello, P., Garcia-Alamino, J., Perera, R., Meats, E., & Glasziou, P. (2006). Self-monitoring of oral anticoagulation: A systematic review and meta-analysis. *Lancet, 367,* 404–411.

Hutchby, I. (2001). Technology, texts, and affordances. *Sociology, 35*(2), 441–456.

Jahns, R.-G. (2014). *8 drivers and barriers that will shape the mhealth app market in the next 5 years*. Available online at: http://research2guidance.com/2014/08/12/8-drivers-and-barriers-which-will-shape-mhealth-market-in-the-next-5-years/. Accessed January 2016.

Kelly, S. (2014). *Apple health has a long way to go, but it's far from hopeless*. Available online at: http://mashable.com/2014/10/08/apple-health-app-needs-work/#YT7aY1PLMGqw. Accessed January 2016.

Logan, A. (2013). Transforming hypertension management using mobile health technology for telemonitoring and self-care support. *Canadian Journal of Cardiology, 29*(5), 579–585.

Logan, A. G., McIsaac, W. J., Tisler, M., Irvine, J., Saunders, A., Dunai, A., et al. (2007). Mobile phone-based remote patient monitoring system for management of hypertension in diabetic patients. *American Journal of Hypertension, 20*(9), 942–948.

Lupton, D. (2013). Quantifying the body: Monitoring and measuring health in the age of mHealth technologies. *Critical Public Health, 23*(4), 393–403.

Lupton, D. (2014a). Critical perspectives on digital health technologies. *Sociology Compass, 8*(12), 1344–1359.

Lupton, D. (2014b). Self-tracking modes: Reflexive self-monitoring and data practices. In: *Imminent citizenships: Personhood and identity politics in the informatic age workshop*. Canberra, ACT, Australia, 27 August.

Lupton, D. (2014c). Apps as artefacts: Towards a critical perspective on mobile health and medical apps. *Societies, 4*(4), 606–622.

May, C., Harrison, R., MacFarlane, A., Williams, T., Mair, F., & Wallace, P. (2003). Why do telemedicine systems fail to normalize as stable models of service delivery? *Journal of Telemedicine and Telecare, 9*, S25–S26.

McMillan, R. (2014, July 29). These medical apps have doctors and the FDA worried. *Wired*. Available online at: http://www.wired.com/2014/07/medical_apps/. Accessed January 2016.

NICE. (2014). NICE recommends self-monitoring tests for people on long-term anticoagulation therapy. Available online at: https://www.nice.org.uk/news/press-and-media/nice-recommends-self-monitoring-tests-for-people-on-long-term-anticoagulation-therapy. Accessed September 2014.

Quinn, P., Habbig, A.-K., Mantovani, E., & De Hert, P. (2013). The data protection and medical device frameworks—Obstacles to the deployment of mHealth across Europe? *European Journal of Health Law,* 185–204.

Snow, C. P. (1961). *Science and government.* Cambridge, MA: Harvard University Press.

Steinhubl, S., Muse, E., & Topol, E. (2013). Can mobile health technologies transform health care? *JAMA, 310*(22), 2395–2396.

Stokes, E. (2012). Nanotechnology and the products of inherited regulation. In A. Faulkner & C. Lawless (Eds.), Material Worlds: Intersections of law, science, technology and society, Special Issue. *Journal of Law and Society, 39*(1), 93–112.

Timmermans, S., & Berg, M. (2003). The practice of medical technology. *Sociology of Health & Illness, 25*(3), 97–114.

Tomlin, Z., Peirce, S., Elwyn, G. & Faulkner, A. (2013). *The adoption space of early-emerging technologies: innovation, evaluation, gatekeeping.* Final research report to Department of Health/NIHR Service Delivery and Organisation Technology Adoption research programme, HMSO. p. 189.

Available online at: http://www.nets.nihr.ac.uk/__data/assets/pdf_file/0014/85100/FR-08-1820-253.pdf. Accessed November 2016.

Ulucanlar, S., Peirce, S., Elwyn, G., & Faulkner, A. (2013). Technology identity: The role of sociotechnical representations in the adoption of medical devices. *Social Science and Medicine, 98,* 95–105.

World Health Organisation. (2014). *mHealth—New horizons for health through mobile technologies.* Global Observatory for eHealth, Vol. 3, p. 6. Geneva, WHO.

10

Commercialising Bodies: Action, Subjectivity and the New Corporate Health Ethic

Christopher Till

Introduction

The focus of this chapter is on the use of particular kinds of commercial personal medical devices (PMDs) which track activity. It will be suggested that these digital self-tracking (DST) devices[1] enable the broad commercialisation of bodies through their transformation of exercise activity into data and their integration of personal wellness activities into corporate structures. While evidence has shown that many users quickly abandon devices (Ledger and McCaffrey 2014), there is still optimism regarding their potential to instigate healthy behaviour change (Campbell 2015) and significant growth in investment in DST, indicating a clear push from corporations (Davies 2015; Field 2014; Statista 2015). The use of corporate wellness (CW) programmes has also increased dramatically in the last few years, especially outside the

C. Till (✉)
Leeds Beckett University, England, UK
e-mail: c.till@leedsbeckett.ac.uk

© The Author(s) 2018
R. Lynch and C. Farrington (eds.), *Quantified Lives and Vital Data*,
Health, Technology and Society, https://doi.org/10.1057/978-1-349-95235-9_10

USA where they are most well-established (BuckConsultants 2014). In addition, there are expected to be 13 million self-tracking devices used in CW by 2018 (ABI search 2013), implemented on the assumption that they will increase productivity through better engagement and motivation at work (Moore and Robinson 2015). These initiatives are attempts by employers to improve the 'wellness' of their employees through the improvement of morale and the creation of a 'culture of health' at work, which, it is proposed, will ultimately increase the 'bottom line' of the employer (GCC, undated b).

CW initiatives have been identified as an effective tool for the transmission of corporate ethics (Conrad and Walsh 1992), and such programmes are considered to be particularly useful in the encouragement of ethics of self-governance (Haunschild 2003; Maravelias 2009), which internalise control mechanisms by making them seem like the choices of individuals (Dale and Burrell 2014). This control is considered to be particularly powerful through its engagement with the self-formation of individuals and the encouragement of blurring of work and non-work tasks and spaces (Conrad 1992; McGillivray 2005). Some scholars have proposed that DST could be consistent with this kind of management ideology due to the prominence of an entrepreneurial disposition of self-improvement in their design (Lupton 2013; Ruckenstein and Pantzar 2015; Whitson 2014).

This chapter will suggest that a conflation between work and health is being achieved through a reorientation of wellness as a topic falling within the remit of employers and as an issue best tackled through management strategies. This will be approached firstly through my reading of two (until recently largely overlooked) philosophers, Guéry and Deleule, to show how the bodies of the population become integrated into the machinery of production. Secondly, I will propose that companies are taking a 'philanthropic' interest in health and well-being that is *not* reducible to the profit motive but which *is* nevertheless inseparable from it. The health of the individual and the health of the economy/organisation are increasingly intertwined, but the definition of health (through a focus on 'wellness') is being aligned with productive capacity. This is happening on both a practical and conceptual level. Practically, the digitisation, accumulation and analysis of bodies through fitness tracking enable the detached management of health and exercise practices. Also, the use of CW programmes encourages the kinds of exercise practices which are conducive to corporate or organisational interests.

The research is based on thematic analysis of nine in-depth interviews conducted with people responsible for implementing or managing digital self-tracking exercise programmes in the UK at large employers, and discourse analysis of promotional material from producers of tracking devices (e.g. *Fitbit*) and providers of wellness programmes (e.g. Global Corporate Challenge, or GCC). All programmes offer forms of digital self-tracking, all used step counts, and some included other forms of exercise. All the initiatives included a competitive element in which participants were arranged into teams who collate their steps together to achieve a goal in a set time period. Several of the initiatives were provided by GCC (GCC, undated a). Some of the other initiatives were developed and maintained by the employers themselves but followed similar models to GCC. Full informed consent to publish verbatim quotations from interviews was given by all research participants.

Productive Bodies

When used personally and for CW programmes, DST devices have the potential to enter into highly intimate relationships with users. Wearable devices integrate with, analyse and potentially affect the biological rhythms of the human body. As with any measurement or analysis, those enabled by these devices only present a partial representation and suggest certain kinds of behaviour as desirable. I suggest that a core, although only partially acknowledged, rationale for these programmes is the generation of 'productive bodies' through engaging the subjectivity of the individual. The conceptualisation of 'productive bodies' is derived from the 1972 book (published in English in 2014) *The Productive Body* by François Guéry and Didier Deleule, and is outlined below.

'Productive bodies' are those which form an efficient and effective cog in the capitalist machine, thus constituting 'the productive body'. This notion (of 'productive bodies' in the plural) is my addition to Guéry and Deleule's conceptual distinction between the biological body (the material body), the social body (the collective population constituted through cooperation) and the productive body (the population that drives and embodies productivity). In order to produce a genuinely productive body (which I suggest is made up of productive bodies), capitalism cannot concern itself merely with the actions and time directly connected with work, but also requires hegemony over the whole productive process. To do this 'it needs to appropriate for itself not only the function of unifying the productive body [...] but also the productive force itself' (Guéry and Deleule 2014, p. 82). What is required, then, is to 'appropriate not the means of production [but] the means of *productivity* or the inner springs of production'. The energy of the working population is thus harnessed through engagement with 'life itself' which comes to be presented as 'productive power' (Guéry and Deleule 2014, p. 106).

It becomes necessary, therefore, for capitalism to engage the entire corporeal and subjective being of the individual. Guéry and Deleule emphasise the role which psychology plays in transforming 'the living machine entirely into efficacious motion' (Guéry and Deleule 2014, p. 112) by short-circuiting the process of reflection and attempting to make desired actions habitual. The most efficient, effective and productive body is that which 'functions without receiving its orders from consciousness [...]. Thus the machine moves by itself' (Guéry and Deleule 2014, p. 115). The central task is, therefore, to enable 'the living machine' to become 'as adapted as possible to the social mechanism into which it is, in fact, integrated, so that that [sic] its productive act develops in optimal conditions and its gears don't grind too loudly' (Guéry and Deleule 2014, p. 118). The productive body requires reactive (not thinking or reflecting) subjects. The habit formation which is central to almost all behaviour change approaches to health (and especially those employing self-tracking) would seem to be a good example of this philosophy.

Contemporary management discourse is suffused with the necessity of engaging the entire subjectivity of the worker in order to maximise their productive output through maintaining engagement (Boltanski and Chiapello 2005), and for some commentators, political economy is becoming identical with 'subjective economy' (Lazzarato 2014: 8).

The subjective focus of management has merged with tactics borrowed from public health, which has resulted in a shift of its gaze from the biomedical to the social and the subjective (Armstrong 1995) through a focus on 'choice', 'personal responsibility' and 'lifestyle' (Armstrong 1993, p. 405; Herrick 2011, p. 3; Larsen 2011, p. 206). The task of public health initiatives has thus become increasingly focused on the enabling of autonomous individuals who can effectively integrate into their social milieu 'in conformity with the demands of neo-liberal democratic structures and values' (Petersen and Lupton 1996, p. 173; Dean 2010)—i.e. the kind of subjects whose 'gears don't grind too loudly'.

The importance of engaging the subjectivity of individual workers in the context of CW is acknowledged by GCC on their website with the assertion that 'people must engage and participate willingly because ultimately only an individual can make the key lifestyle changes required to improve their physical and mental health' (GCC, undated c). Engagement is seen to be the key factor in achieving wellness but is always tied to profitability for the company, as a GCC report asserts:

> The data shows that employees with the highest engagement levels also reported feeling more productive [...] In other words, those who were connected with their workplaces reported better outputs. (GCC 2016a)

In the contemporary economy in which productivity is dependent on affective skills, creativity and symbolic manipulation, and with workers demanding autonomy from stifling bureaucratic structures, it is above all through engagement that workers are integrated within the machinery of capitalism. The 'means of productivity' and the 'productive power' (Guéry and Deleule 2014, p. 106) which capitalism must appropriate is no longer just physical capacities (as for Marx) or the psyche (as it was for Guéry and Deleule) but now includes the affective lives of the workers. This can be seen through the interest GCC shows in happiness:

> [E]ven though the reason someone is happy may have nothing to do with the workplace, research shows that happier workers are better liked and often out-perform their less happy colleagues.

> They stay with their employers for longer, have fewer sick days, are more punctual and more likely to contribute beyond the requirements of their job. Given the evidence, work is an appropriate place to start the conversation about happiness. (GCC 2016b, p. 5)

Although the significance of happiness for productivity can be traced at least back to early twentieth-century management gurus Frederick Winslow Taylor and Elton Mayo (Cederström and Spicer 2015, p. 73), the technical approach and behaviourist philosophy make the current approach distinctive. Happiness is shrunk to a phenomenon which can be enabled through management strategies and 'nudges' from electronic devices as 'that's essentially what happiness is: a healthy habit' (GCC 2016b, p. 7). Crucially, these happiness habits are enabled by cultural not structural factors. But this is a particular way of understanding culture, as something transmitted like a virus through a collection of monadic individuals. This can be seen in the assertion that the way in which employers can enable workers to be happy is through their own disposition and enabling 'positive emotional contagion' (GCC 2016b, p. 7). In this model, happiness is something which can be 'caught' from others but is only made possible through individualised strategies:

> We often get so busy that we neglect the things that bring us joy, we forget self-care. The irony is that we're doing it to be more productive. Yet when we prioritise self- care, and positivity within that, we become happier and more productive. (GCC 2016b, p. 10)

William Davies interprets this incorporation of happiness into the productive process as a utilitarian understanding of emotion, in which it is seen as a source of energy which is valued only when it is 'directed towards goals other than being happy' (Davies 2016, p. 115) rather than as an intrinsic good in itself. Happiness is thus a force which is outside capitalist enterprise but is valued only when channelled in such a way as to increase productive intensity. In the contemporary workplace, happiness, self-realisation and authenticity take on an ideological character, presenting an ideal worker defined through their happiness and productivity (Cederström and Grassman 2010, pp. 111, 120–122).

Workers are encouraged to identify with this ideal which is nevertheless always out of their reach, and through this become subject to discipline and control through affective investment in securing a happier and more balanced life (Bloom 2016, p. 600).

Through behavioural tactics and automated prompts and reminders, the devices and programmes discussed in this chapter attempt to constitute a reactive subject smoothly integrated with their productive context. The qualities and behaviours which are encouraged are those which enable the integration of bodies into capital accumulation rather than those associated with health per se. Intervention through these means enables corporations and organisations to fulfil their aims of doing social good through constituting healthy subjects while creating conditions for greater productivity.

Philanthrocapitalism

While the constitution of well-integrated, 'productive bodies' is necessary for productivity, this cannot simply be achieved through authoritarian commands for individuals to fall in line with the demands of capitalism. Rather, the practices of capital accumulation must be integrated with an ethical calling (Weber 2001). I claim that one aim of CW DST initiatives is the instantiation of a productive ethic through the encouragement of practices of self-assessment and management. The companies involved in selling DST devices and using them for wellness programmes both have a genuine interest in the well-being of the public and feel a responsibility to make a positive impact upon it. However, they expect to do this while further enhancing productivity and broader capitalist interests. For this reason, I suggest that they are engaged in a form of 'philanthrocapitalism', which has been defined as:

> the idea that capitalism is or can be charitable in and of itself. The claim is that capitalist mechanisms are superior to all others (especially the state) when it comes to not only creating economic but also human progress; that the market and market actors are or should be made the prime creators of the good society. (Thorup 2013, p. 556)

Thorup (2013 p. 558) builds on Boltanski and Chiappelo (2005) to suggest that 'philanthrocapitalism' is one of the key ways in which contemporary ethical critiques of capitalism are integrated into its practices and become a strength of capitalism. Philanthropy is not something which happens outside business hours or in addition to commercial activity; rather, it is part of 'competitiveness planning' and the capitalist enterprise itself comes to be seen as philanthropic (Thorup 2013, p. 563).

I suggest that an analogous situation is emerging in the field of health and (particularly) exercise. Corporations increasingly see it as their role to improve the health and wellness of the population (i.e., not only their employees). This general tendency can be seen in a research report produced by the organisation 'Business for Social Responsibility', who found that:

> …companies face increasing pressure to improve health outcomes by promoting wellness and prevention—not only for their employees, but for the broader population that is impacted by corporate actions. Stakeholders from employees, government, community organizations, consumers, and investors recognize that private sector action [...] reflects a sphere of influence that extends well beyond a company's core employee base. (BSR 2013, p. 5)

The report also suggests that increasingly employees want to work for companies who demonstrate that they care for their employees (BSR 2013). Crucially, companies consider their philanthropic activities to be commensurate with their organisational goals and usually consider the best route to achieving them to be through 'responsibilising' the individual (Thorup 2013: 561). This alignment of management strategy with the values of workers was clearly a driving factor for the participants in this study. As one HR worker asserted:

> From our perspective it was very much [...] advertised as a staff benefit [...] on a larger scale it attracts employees to the [organisation] and retains them once they're here [...] Alongside that it also has additional benefits some go towards the efficiency of the university itself including

the amount of carbon produced and also perhaps things such as increased levels of motivation amongst employees and others are far more individual such as weight loss, healthy habits being implemented into everyday life for the employees.

The CW programme at this organisation was paid for out of a carbon reduction fund and was considered to be an effective means of reconciling management concerns for productivity with staff desires to improve their health along with broader environmental strategies. All three of these can be interpreted as ethical projects which are neatly combined through technological disciplining of individuals. Another participant working as an HR manager assessed the success of their initiatives through analysis of responses in their staff survey, which measured to what extent the organisation was perceived to care about the well-being of employees. They made sense of their high scores on this measure as being due to the simple fact that initiatives are offered to employees, rather than their objective outcomes in terms of behaviour change or health benefits:

> I think the reason that we are higher [...] isn't because we've got lots of people participating in these things. I think they just know that it's there and it gives them a good feeling about working for an employer that does these things even if they choose not to participate.

This 'good feeling' is seen as central to motivating workers in the contemporary economy, as a 'thought piece' published by the UK government backing employee engagement task force 'Engage for Success' states:

> People are seeking something more meaningful and sustainable than engaging with a corporate strategy. Many employees want to engage with social missions beyond the organisation. (Sparrow 2014: unpaged)

Health and environmental improvement are seen as the kinds of goals which provide workers with the motivation to improve productivity by infusing work with meaning beyond immediate organisational concerns. One participant summarised their organisation's motivation for instigating the DST programme as being:

a healthy workforce but it was engagement, the whole staff engagement thing as well. The feedback we got from the people who did was, aside from some of the competitiveness, it was more of a real team spirit and there was a buzz in the air.

GCC uses the potential for their programmes to boost engagement as one of their key selling points. Similarly to the comments from participants above, it is not necessarily individual behaviour or concrete health outcomes that are significant; rather, 'culture' is the target. They suggest that:

> Cultures that promote wellbeing, safety and human connection drive engagement and ultimately become more competitive. GCC Insights data shows that healthy, engaged employees are productive employees. Employee engagement may be intrinsic, but employers can create a culture that connects it to better business outcomes. (GCC 2016a, p. 7)

DST initiatives are seen as a means to encourage engagement and 're-energise' teams (GCC 2016a, p. 10), increasing productivity both through disciplining workers into productive practices and, perhaps more significantly, making them *feel* better about their workplace and themselves. This latter affective force is essential for the maximisation of productivity in contemporary capitalism (Berardi 2009; Lazzarato 2014).

When companies are discussed as philanthrocapitalist this is usually due to their charitable giving, which does not apply to the context explored here. Instead, I refer to the tactics which companies use to construct themselves as 'a self-avowed socially-conscious, forward-thinking corporate citizen' (Giardina 2010, p. 135) and in so doing claim an area of social life as legitimately within their remit. Crucially, it is strategies of (or associated with) capitalist accumulation which are presented as the most effective means of achieving a social good—in this context, improved wellness. Philanthrocapitalism is driven by 'the desire to bring "hard-nosed" strategy [and] performance' (McGoey 2014, p. 111) to philanthropy. As will be demonstrated below, business strategies (focused on productivity) and an emphasis on performance metrics are central to self-tracking approaches to health and especially those implemented as part of wellness schemes.

Activity

The philanthrocapitalist intervention of corporations and organisations into the intimate lives of individuals is primarily predicated not on the improvement of health as such but on the increase in activity. This can be seen in the focus on the reduction in sedentarism and the emphasis on devices and initiatives built around walking and running, as exemplified by the slogan of Global Corporate Challenge: 'Get The World Moving'. It has previously been noted that the practices of self-reflection and optimisation associated with ST are consistent with neoliberal ideology and an entrepreneurial disposition towards the self (Lupton 2013; Ruckenstein and Pantzar 2015). Central to the constitution of the subject of neoliberal governmentality—in Foucault's (2008, pp. 231–232) analysis—is 'human capital theory', which is based on the 'managerialization of personal identity' and the 'capitalization of the meaning of life' (Gordon cited in Bröckling 2016, p. 27). But in order for this to occur, 'life' needs to be formulated in such a way that 'capitalization' is possible. In practice, this means that it is made equivalent and comparable. In the contemporary form of capitalism:

> the general equivalent - what the status of persons and things is measured by - is *activity*…[which] surmounts the oppositions between work and non-work, the stable and the unstable, wage earning and non-wage-earning class, paid work and voluntary work. (Boltanksi and Chiapello 2005, p. 109)

'Activity' for Boltanski and Chiapello has become a generic measure of virtuous behaviour; 'activity' is a good in and of itself. Similarly, Stephan Lessenich has proposed that the promotion of 'activity' is the primary organising principle of contemporary capitalism (Dörre et al. 2015) which can also be observed in the often identified 'cult of busyness' (Ehrenreich 1985; Robinson and Godbey 2005). This means that capitalist enterprises promote 'activity' as an inherently virtuous category only partly because of its connection to productivity. For Muriel Gillick, walking and running are now seen as inherently personal and social goods and as the marker of general wellness, which are considered unproblematically virtuous activities (Gillick 1984, p. 381). This point highlights not only the well-worn insight that health and fitness have long been associated with morality but also explains the widespread uptake of a particular activity (running) through its seemingly natural alignment with personal and social virtue, which has only increased since Gillick's article was published in 1984. Therefore, when employers and corporations become dedicated to encouraging individuals to engage in running or walking, this may help to put their actions beyond potential critique. 'Activity', through its reconstitution as a virtuous activity, has become simply 'good practice' inside and outside the workplace.

It is my suggestion that DST devices and CW programmes using such technologies function to constitute productive bodies while achieving social 'goods' in a manner consistent with capitalist enterprise, and that the main way in which this is done is through the promotion of 'activity'. A function of corporate wellness initiatives is to conflate work and non-work life and practices (McGillivray 2005, p. 125; Holliday and Thompson 2001, p. 125), in particular through transforming the workplace into a 'health-promoting setting' (Chu et al. 1997, p. 381). The developments discussed here represent a more specific intensification of this process. Rather than working from the assumption that 'a healthy worker is a good worker', it suggests that 'activity' is inherently good for work and health.

Activity is perceived as inherently good for all, but in order to avoid negative consequences, it must be directed in a productive way. The balance between 'disengagement' (or lack of activity) and 'burnout' (from being overactive) has become one of the main concerns of human resource management (Dagher et al. 2015; Maslach and Leiter 2008; Saks 2006; Wollard and Shuck 2011). Interview respondents in my study placed great emphasis on the ability of CW DST programmes to encourage and stimulate activity. As one occupational therapist responsible for implementing such an initiative stated:

Our key aim was to have an impact mainly on sedentary roles but also recognising as well that we could have the busiest of people like for example porters or nurses who are on their feet all the time but they'll go home and do absolutely nothing. So I suppose we tried to look at it quite holistically but the other thing for us as well was more about engaging with the people who didn't do things.

The focus for this respondent was clearly on increasing activity even for those occupying highly active roles at work. For many of the respondents, the programmes were not just useful in encouraging physical activity, but were also part of stimulating broader engagement. In particular, greater social interaction (particularly between workers who did not usually engage with one another) was seen as a major benefit. Friendly rivalry and teamwork were considered to be a fundamental aspect of the initiatives, which was inspired by the sharing of achievements via social media. The automated digitisation of activity in all kinds of DST makes comparison and sharing with others particularly easy and has led some to suggest that self-tracking is an inherently communicative phenomenon (Lomborg and Frandsen 2015).

One organisation which developed a walking challenge app with the help of an external company built their whole strategy around 'activity':

we put together the "active staff" programme which has different strands, one strand of "active staff" being [...] our large scale challenges and events including our walking challenges. [...] Another aspect of our programme is "active sites" [...] We have our "live active" [...] which is a GP exercise referral scheme which runs across [local health authority] that is a referral from your GP practice to a physiotherapist but as a part of the "active staff" programme we are currently piloting a self-referral pathway so the idea is that staff can access the "live active" service, which is a one-to-one intervention for behavioural change support.

'Activity' and being 'active' are here thoroughly integrated across the whole approach to workplace wellness. This emphasis on increasing activity is mirrored in the advice provided by *Fitbit* on their website:

Doing the dishes? Multitask when you stand at the sink and load the dishwasher. Do calf raises while rinsing, and pause to do a squat for every plate, bowl, or glass you put in the machine.

Go upstairs, again. Doing a chore that requires your presence on the second floor? Slip in an extra flight on your way there, by walking up, immediately turning around to go down, and walking up again. (Farrell 2015)

This advice is not directly connected to the tracking devices which *Fitbit* sell; rather, they have an interest in increasing activity more broadly. This advice can be read as simply part of the advertising strategy to bring readers to their site and demonstrate their caring credentials. I, however, am less interested in their genuine motivations (if such things can be determined) than the fact that they see such an interest in the health of people in general as within their realm of responsibility or concern. Companies such as *Fitbit* see the improvement of health, through the promotion of activity, as part of their mission.

It is also through activity that the work and health contexts are brought together. On their website *Fitbit* articulate the convergence of exercise and work through advertising copy for their *Surge* wristband:

Work hard.

But, also, work better.

Designed with advanced smartwatch features, Surge lets you run your day, your way. Text and call notifications keep you on your game throughout the day, while music control helps you find the motivation you need to prepare for a big meeting or beat your best in a big race. (Fitbit, undated)

The motivational phrasing can be applied to exercise or work:

See what you've done, then do more. Surge automatically and wirelessly syncs to your computer and 120 + leading smartphones—showing your stats as detailed charts and graphs—so you can access your progress anywhere. (Fitbit, undated)

Using the kinds of technologies currently available, movement is much easier to track than other forms of wellness-promoting behaviour; as such, it is becoming one of the key organising principles of contemporary capitalism. This is because it is useful for increasing the productivity of workers (for directly generating income through sales of devices and the production of valuable data), in addition to the virtuous aura which justifies the spread of capitalist logics to increasing areas of life.

Activity is here presented as beneficial for the improvement of health and productivity. The promotion of activity by corporations is thus deemed to be a social good in itself, as it will increase the health and well-being of the individuals who engage in it at the same time that it helps those individuals to be more productive at work. The promotion of activity is also useful for the producers of DST and employers who implement them as part of wellness activities. The former benefit from the generation of valuable data and the latter from a more productive and engaged workforce. While there are other means through which to achieve health and wellness, these devices and initiatives are helping to constitute an increasing alignment between activity, morality and health.

Conclusion

Digital technologies perhaps integrate the bodies of the population into the machinery of capitalism more completely than at any other time in history. This is achieved so comprehensively because it is accomplished through merging the goals of the organisation with people's everyday lives. Undoubtedly, this means that companies are more ethical (in the sense that they are engaged with ethical practice), but does not mean that they are any less engaged in the process of formulating social relations for the purposes of profitability. Capital accumulation and ethical practice have merged in contemporary capitalism; what is good for the company and what is good for society have come to be seen as the same thing. As Boltanski and Chiappelo (2005) show, the critiques of capitalism which it integrates into its functioning are a vital part of the legitimation process. But when capitalism seeks to make itself more ethical, it does not leave the object of its ethical attentions untouched. Rather, just as capitalist enterprise is reformed through engagement with critique, so is that which it seeks to improve in society. What has been shown here is that attempts by corporations and organisations to improve the health of the public and employees reconstitute health in terms which are useful for capitalism. Principally, health is redefined in terms of activity and engagement with others; healthy bodies become synonymous with productive bodies.

The emphasis on activity for producing health is partly due to the existing capacities of tracking technologies; they can monitor particular kinds of movement (such as running and walking) in a much more obviously meaningful way than, for instance, meditation. Manufacturers of PMDs used for self-tracking and those designing and implementing CW programmes draw explicit connections between exercise activity and productivity, with the same devices being positioned as able to improve both. This is perhaps not surprising given that information technologies (which DSTs can be classified as) were initially principally designed as a means for the control of workflow (van Dijk 2006). When technologies and management systems built for the maximisation of productivity are applied to exercise, it makes sense that the latter will start to seem more like work. Employers and corporations have shown a growing interest in promoting exercise activity as a moral good. Simultaneously, digital technologies such as PMDs have enabled the kinds of measurement, standardisation and incentivisation often associated with work to seep into everyday lives (Till 2014). In the process, health and exercise are coming to be judged in terms of productivity, and work is being presented as a means of achieving wellness and self-fulfilment. Work and non-work seem to be blurring with productivity, which is increasingly the key measure of both.

Note

1. DSTs use accelerometers to measure the acceleration of forces and are central to self-tracking activities and culture as they are the main proxy used when counting the amount of steps taken or energy expended (Swan 2009: 510).

Acknowledgements All interview material used in this chapter was gained with informed consent and is used with permission.

References

ABIresearch. (2013). *Corporate Wellness is a 13 Million Unit Wearable Wireless Device Opportunity*. 25 September 2013. Available at: https://www.abiresearch.com/press/corporate-wellness-is-a-13-million-unit-wearable-w/ [Accessed on October 12, 2015].

Armstrong, D. (1993). Public health spaces and the fabrication of identity. *Sociology, 27*(3), 393–410.

Armstrong, D. (1995). The rise of surveillance medicine. *Sociology of Health & Illness, 17*(3), 393–404.

Berardi, F. (2009). *The Soul at work: From alienation to autonomy*. Semiotext(e): Los Angeles.

Bloom, P. (2016). Work as the contemporary limit of life: Capitalism, the death drive, and the lethal fantasy of 'work-life balance'. *Organization, 23*(4), 588–606.

Boltanski, L., & Chiapello, E. (2005). *The new spirit of capitalism*. London: Verso.

Bröckling, U. (2016). *The entrepreneurial self: Fabricating a new type of subject*. London: Sage.

BSR. (2013). *A new CSR frontier: Business and population health: Mobilizing CSR to strengthen corporate engagement on health and wellness across the value chain*. Available at: http://www.bsr.org/reports/BSR_A_New_CSR_Frontier_Business_and_Population_Health.pdf [Accessed on April 10, 2016].

BuckConsultants. (2014). *Working Well: A Global Survey of Health Promotion, Workplace Wellness, and Productivity Strategies*. Available at: https://www.bucksurveys.com/BuckSurveys/Portals/0/aspdnsf/BuckSurveys_OrdersDownload/Health%20and%20Productivity/GW_Exec_Summary_Global.pdf [Accessed on January 07, 2016].

Caffentzis, G. (undated). *The work/energy crisis and the apocalypse*. Available at: https://libcom.org/library/workenergy-crisis-apocalypse-george-caffentzis [Accessed on April 10, 2016].

Campbell, D. (2015). Prof Bruce Keogh: Wearable technology plays a crucial part in NHS future. *The Guardian*, 19 January 2015. Available at: http://www.theguardian.com/society/2015/jan/19/prof-bruce-keogh-wearable-technology-plays-crucial-part-nhs-future [Accessed on September 09, 2015].

Cederström, C., & Grassman, R. (2010). The unbearable weight of happiness. In C. Cederström & C. Hoedemakers (Eds.), *Lacan and organization* (pp. 101–132). London: MayFlyBooks.

Cederström, C., & Spicer, A. (2015). *The wellness syndrome*. Cambridge: Polity.

Chu, C., Driscoll, T., & Dwyer, S. (1997). The health-promoting workplace: An integrative perspective. *Australian and New Zealand Journal of Public Health, 21*(4), 377–385.

Conrad, P., & Walsh, D. C. (1992). The new corporate health ethic: Lifestyle and the social control of work. *International Journal of Health Services Research, 22*(1), 89–111.

Dagher, G., Chapa, O., & Junaid, N. (2015). The historical evolution of employee engagement and self-efficacy constructs. *Journal of Management History, 21*(2), 232–256.

Dale, K., & Burrell, G. (2014). Being occupied: An embodied re-reading of organizational "wellness". *Organization, 21*(2), 159–177.

Davies, S. (2015). Wearable tech usage to grow by 60 Percent this year. *Bionicly,* 3 November 2015. Available at: http://bionicly.com/wearable-tech-growth-emarketer/ [Accessed November 4, 2015].

Davies, W. (2016). *The Happiness industry: How the government and big business sold us well-being*. London: Verso.

Dean, M. (2010). *Governmentality: Power and rule in modern society*. London: Sage.

Ehrenreich, B. (1985, February 21). Hers. *The New York Times,* Available at:http://www.forbes.com/sites/dell/2012/05/17/managing-distraction-beware-the-cult-of-busyness/ [Accessed January 5, 2016].

Dörre, K., Lessenich, S., & Rosa, H. (2015). *Sociology, capitalism, critique*. London: Verso.

Farrell, K. D. (2015). 8 Crazy-Simple Ways Parents Can Slip Fitness into Their Day. *The Fitbit Blog.* Available at: https://blog.fitbit.com/8-crazy-simple-ways-parents-can-slip-fitness-into-their-day-2/ [Accessed April 24, 2016].

Field, A. (2014). Venture Capital Flocks to the 'Quantified Self'. *The network: Cisco's Technology News Site*, 3 June 2014. Available at: http://newsroom.cisco.com/feature-content?type=webcontent&articleId=1425860 [Accessed November 10, 2015].

Fitbit. (undated). Train smarter. Go farther. *Fitbit.com* Available at: https://www.fitbit.com/uk/surge [Accessed January 7, 2016].

Foucault, M. (2008). *The birth of biopolitics: Lectures at the Collège de France, 1978–1979*. Houndmills, Basingstoke: Palgrave Macmillan.

Giardina, M. (2010). One day, one goal? PUMA, corporate philanthropy and the cultural politics of brand 'Africa'. *Sport in Society: Cultures, Commerce, Media, Politics, 13*(1), 130–142.

Gillick, M. (1984). Health promotion, jogging, and the pursuit of the moral life. *Journal of Health Politics, Policy and Law, 9*(3), 369–387.

GCC. (undated a). GCC. *gettheworldmoving.com* Available at: https://www.gettheworldmoving.com/ [Accessed April 10, 2016].

GCC. (undated b). Proof it works. *gettheworldmoving.com* Available at: https://www.gettheworldmoving.com/proof-it-works [Accessed April 10, 2016].

GCC. (undated c). How it works. *gettheworldmoving.com* Available at: https://www.gettheworldmoving.com/how-it-works [Accessed April 10, 2016].

GCC. (2016a). Get Engaged: How a healthy culture can drive greater employee commitment and engagement. *GCC Insights.* Available at: http://info.gettheworldmoving.com/engaged-employees.html?utm_source=resourcespage&utm_medium=website&utm_campaign=engagement [Accessed September 16, 2016].

GCC. (2016b). Happy days: Drive better business outcomes with happiness and positive emotion. *GCC Insights.* Available at: http://info.gettheworldmoving.com/happiness-at-work-US.html?utm_source=homepage&utm_medium=website&utm_campaign=happiness [Accessed September 16, 2016].

Guéry, F., & Deleule, D. (2014). *The productive body.* Winchester: Zero Books.

Haunschild, A. (2003). Humanization through discipline? Foucault and the goodness of employee health programmes. *Journal of Critical Postmodern Organization Science, 2*(3), 46–59.

Herrick, C. (2011). *Governing health and consumption: Sensible citizens, behaviour and the city.* Bristol: The Policy Press.

Holliday, R., & Thompson, G. (2001). A body of work. In R. Holliday & J. Hassard (Eds.), *Contested bodies.* London: Routledge.

Larsen, L. T. (2011). The Birth of lifestyle politics: The biopolitical management of lifestyle diseases in the United States and Denmark. In U. Bröckling, S. Krasmann, & T. Lemke (Eds.), *Governmentality: Current issues and future challenges* (pp. 201–220). London: Routledge.

Lazzarato, M. (2014). *Signs and machines: Capitalism and the production of subjectivity.* Semiotext(e): Los Angeles.

Ledger, D., & McCaffrey, D. (2014). *Inside wearables: How the science of human behaviour change offers the secret to long-term engagement.* Endeavour Partners. Available at: http://endeavourpartners.net/assets/Endeavour-Partners-Wearables-and-the-Science-of-Human-Behavior-Change-Part-1-January-20141.pdf [Accessed January 2, 2016].

Lomborg, S., & Frandsen, K. (2015). Self-tracking as communication. *Information, Communication & Society*. doi:10.1080/1369118X.2015.1067710.

Lupton, D. (2013). Understanding the human machine. *IEEE Technology and Society Magazine, 32,* 25–30.

Maravelias, C. (2009). Health promotion and flexibility: Extending and obscuring power in organizations. *British Journal of Management* 20(S), 194–203.

Maslach, C., & Leiter, M. P. (2008). Early predictors of job burnout and engagement. *Journal of Applied Psychology, 93*(3), 498–512.

McGillivray, D. (2005). Fitter, happier, more productive: Governing working bodies through wellness. *Culture and Organization, 11*(2), 125–138.

McGoey, L. (2014). The philanthropic state: Market-state hybrids in the philanthrocapitalist turn. *Third World Quarterly, 35*(1), 109–125.

Moore, P., & Robinson, A. (2015). The quantified self: What counts in the neo-liberal workplace. *New Media & Society*. doi:10.1177/146/4448/5604328.

Petersen, A., & Lupton, D. (1996). *The new public health: Health and self in the age of risk*. London: Sage.

Robinson, J., & Godbey, G. (2005). Business as usual. *Social Research: An International Quarterly, 72*(2), 407–426.

Ruckenstein, M., & Pantzar, M. (2015). Beyond the quantified self: Thematic exploration of a dataistic paradigm. *New Media & Society*. doi:10.1177/1461444815609081.

Saks, A. M. (2006). Antecedents and consequences of employee engagement. *Journal of Managerial Psychology, 21*(7), 600–619.

Sparrow, P. (2014). *Are we now mature enough to ask the harder questions, the 'engage with what?' challenge*. Engage For Success. Available at: http://engageforsuccess.org/wp-content/uploads/2015/09/Paul-Sparrow.pdf [Accessed September 16, 2016].

Statista. (2015). Facts and statistics on wearable technology. *Statista*. Available at: http://www.statista.com/topics/1556/wearable-technology/ [Accessed January 1, 2016].

Swan, M. (2009). Emerging patient-driven health care models: An examination of health social networks, consumer personalized medicine and quantified self-tracking. *International Journal of Environmental Research and Public Health, 6*(2), 492–525.

Thorup, M. (2013). Pro Bono? On philanthrocapitalism as ideological answer to inequality. *Ephemera: Theory & Politics Organization, 13*(3), 555–576.

Till, C. (2014). Exercise as labour: Quantified self and the transformation of exercise into labour. *Societies, 4*(3), 446–462.

van Dijk, J. (2006). *The network society: Social aspects of new media.* London: Sage.

Weber, M. (2001). *The Protestant ethic and the spirit of capitalism.* London: Routledge.

Whitson, J. (2014). Foucault's fitbit: Governance and gamification. In S. P. Walz & S. Deterding (Eds.), *The gameful world: Approaches, issues and applications* (pp. 339–358). Cambridge, Mass: MIT Press.

Wollard, K., & Shuck, B. (2011). Antecedents to employee engagement: A structured review of the literature. *Advances in Developing Human Resources, 13*(4), 429–446.

11

Co-Designing for Care: Craft and Wearable Wellbeing

Anthony Kent and Peta Bush

Introduction

This chapter examines a neglected aspect of personal medical devices (PMDs) as products of complex design processes that function at the intersection between aesthetic and scientific agendas. Whilst these intersections have been the subject of considerable discussion since Simon's (1969) seminal work on design and creativity, the personal element of medical devices highlights more recent developments in design thinking about the relationship between designer, object and user. One approach that has gained significance in recent years has been participative design, in which users are brought into the design process to contribute to the designed outcome. In medical contexts, patients have tended to be the

A. Kent (✉)
Nottingham Trent University, Nottingham, UK
e-mail: anthony.kent@ntu.ac.uk

P. Bush (✉)
London Metropolitan University, London, UK
e-mail: bushp@staff.londonmet.ac.uk

© The Author(s) 2018
R. Lynch and C. Farrington (eds.), *Quantified Lives and Vital Data*,
Health, Technology and Society, https://doi.org/10.1057/978-1-349-95235-9_11

passive recipients of designed objects and services, with limited engagement in creating a user-centred functionality and aesthetic. However, engagement in the design of medical devices may have positive effects on user motivations to adherence. As such, a better and more inclusive design of PMDs may improve their use and ultimately result in better health. To demonstrate this as a possibility, a case study of participatory design is presented, in which a medical device is conceptualised as jewellery. Participant involvement in the design of an attractive and personally meaningful product met participants' desire for more personalised solutions, greater empowerment and enhanced sense of wellbeing. Through situating this case study in relation to design practices and theory, including the design process and 'good' design and how meaning is made through design, we open up a new approach to PMDs and medical technology, emphasising the importance of considering design. Building on this perspective, we suggest that through a co-design process PMDs might be made more personalised, and that we might find ways in which PMDs, and other health technologies, could be better designed for care through design collaborations.

Good design is essential to both appearance and performance of products. When they are easier to use, fit for purpose and attractive, they have motivational qualities; the idea of "I want to use it" rather than "I have to use it" invests a degree of ownership in the designed device. However, design refers to both the process and outcome of the activity (Walsh, 1996) and the route to participatory design is an evolutionary one. Explaining design, and what designers do, defines the possibilities for patient engagement through designer problem-solving, 'know-how' and the designed outcomes. When design practices combine with an increasing awareness of the importance of person-centred healthcare, they form a compelling focus for research (Golubnitschaja et al. 2014).

The argument is extended by the US National Institutes of Health. In order to balance cost reduction with improvements to health and healthcare, they proposed that medicine should move away from "one size fits all" therapies to become more predictive, pre-emptive, personalised and participative over time (National Institutes of Health 2008). The development of service and interaction design and the proliferation of sophisticated yet affordable PMDs facilitate this approach. Some personalised devices (e.g. glasses and hearing aids) have been used for many years, but they increasingly include more complex technologies (e.g. blood pressure monitors) that enable patients to independently monitor their own health. Such devices clearly provide opportunities to gather and communicate personal information. However, it is less clear how the appearance, functionality or symbolic meaning of technologies contribute to personalisation and individualised experiences.

Within this spectrum of devices, the provision of personal orthotics presents a particular challenge. The correct supply and fit of orthotic devices can be a major factor in the management of a health condition and in preventative care (HEC 2009). These are addressed by NHS England's (2015) guidance for understanding patients' needs and the recommendation of a ten-step process. Whilst most of these steps focus on service provision and transformation, others focus on patients and devices and include the need for devices to be comfortable and provide appropriate support and accurate fit, a choice of high-quality providers, and the need to be cosmetically acceptable, in particular for image-sensitive younger people. These guidelines point towards a significant change for orthosis provision that improves both patient satisfaction and adherence.

Since orthotics are orthopaedic devices for immobilization, restraint or support of the body (Glanze et al. 1990), personalisation is required to offer the close fit necessary for them to function appropriately, and to allow people to feel an emotional attachment towards them, as they would towards other worn objects or 'wearables' that match their sense of fashion or style. Therapeutic user engagement addresses this challenge through opportunities to develop craft techniques for personalisation and, in so doing, highlights the relationship between designers and users, design practices and design thinking.

The crafting of splints in particular has a long historical connection. Twentieth-century European wars provided the catalyst for the development of both materials and techniques. In the First World War, sculptors and woodcarvers applied craft sensibilities to explore the use of materials such as papier-mâché, leather and textiles, developing new forms of fabrication (Llewellyn 2010). During the Second World War, furniture designers Eames applied their plywood-forming technology to leg-splint design, further demonstrating how the crafting of materials, methods and anatomical knowledge has contributed to personalised, well-fitting devices. And whilst craft has influenced splint-making, so the process of splint-making has also influenced craft and design culture (Pullin 2009).

The personalisation of orthotic devices, the use of craft techniques and interactive design principles may create a new model for developing effective treatments. Our case study demonstrates how participants with Ehlers–Danlos Syndrome-hypermobility type (EDS-ht)[1]—a condition which requires the use of splints—felt about wearing conventional splints, and how engagement in the design of different splints enabled them to create better-fitting and more personally meaningful devices. In order to explore a design approach to PMDs, we first situate PMDs within design theory, drawing on ideas of what constitutes 'good' design, how meaning is made through design, interactive approaches, and how it might be possible to design for care.

Design

The development of orthotics demonstrates how design processes and outcomes themselves are subject to change both in activity and interpretation. Reflecting on the development of design, Buchanan (2001) describes places or placements as areas of discovery and invention that characterise the practice of design. They demonstrate new 'orders' of practice and research as a way to answer new project and societal demands. Buchanan argues that design's trajectory has moved from 'symbols' (graphic and communication design) to 'things' (product design), 'interactions' (interaction design) and finally 'systems' (environment and system design). These orders are not rigidly fixed, but represent the growing scale and complexity of design interventions. The definition of design that emerges is by no means straightforward but necessarily captures the relationship between the creative process and realised solution as 'the intentional solution of a problem, by the creation of plans for a new sort of thing' (Parsons 2016, p. 11). In this, design distinguishes itself from craft, which draws on the development of traditional skills and the application of standard rules to materials (Parsons 2016).

From an object perspective, PMDs can be considered as designed products that demonstrate a relationship between form and function. Functionalist approaches developed the principles of functional aesthetics, emphasising geometry, precision, simplicity and economy in the design of products. Design should be from the 'inside out' so that the form of a product follows from its function, an approach later summarised by Mies van der Rohe, one of modernism's leading proponents, as 'less is more'. Arguably, in this tradition, functional form was realised as a styling feature, a fashion for nothing, much as other movements were associated with style through different forms of ornamentation (Lambert 1993). In contrast to this minimal European approach, styling features were very much a part of mid-twentieth-century American modernist design. These designers emphasised the product's exterior in response to commercial demands for the creation of product appeal. Raymond Loewy famously pronounced that 'ugliness does not sell' and created streamlined styles favouring non-functional, aerodynamic shapes—an approach that remained influential to the 1960s (Ulrich and Eppinger 2012). However, a defining feature of both approaches is their concern with new materials and, with them, new possibilities for design.

Good design came to be explicitly stated in another way, through the practices of industrial design and new product development (NPD). Of enduring influence are Dreyfus's (1967) five critical goals to achieve utility, appearance, ease of maintenance, low costs and communication, in which the visual quality of products communicates corporate design philosophy and mission. In this way, industrial product design came to be considered in two important dimensions: first, ergonomics, which encompasses all aspects of a product that relate to its human interfaces, and includes novelty of interaction needs, maintenance and safety issues; and second, aesthetics, considerations of whether visual product differentiation is required and the importance of pride of ownership, image and fashion (Ulrich and Eppinger 2012). This approach advanced consideration of the user and user needs in respect of products, albeit defined by the designer and the organisational environment.

Meaning-Making Through Design

Whilst PMDs can be considered within the product order, the expansion of design into a broader problem-solving activity is reflected in the possibilities of approaches that consider design in terms of meaning (Brown 2008). With these approaches, objects are shaped by human intentionality and human-made things are dependent on intentions to exist, and thus part of the language that design can create and shape.

Krippendorff's philosophical and semantic approach defines design and designers' work as a matter of creating meaning rather than artefacts (Krippendorff 1989, 2006). In this account, meaning is a cognitively constructed relationship that selectively connects features of an object and features of its context into a coherent unity. Objects must always be seen in contexts of other things, situations and users, including the observer themselves. Thus, meaning not only signifies a product's basic functions and aesthetics, but also carries an emotional and symbolic value, bringing a product message to the user (Krippendorff 2006). In PMD contexts, it is pertinent to consider design as making sense of things: people and very personal items, their relationship to who gave them, and reminders of the giver. Wheelchair design, for example, offers the opportunity to explain design-inspired innovation, meaning and how design systems functions. In the design process, the wheelchair can be thought of as an extension of the self and a means of self-expression, as a physical object but one with implicit messages. The product not only signifies its basic functions and aesthetics but also carries an emotional and symbolic value with a set of symbolic meanings for both the user and individuals observing its use. The product acts as an extension of the human body and mind by giving the user both independence and identity. Design is important as it allows for new perspectives from the beginning and through the whole process of product development (Utterback et al. 2006).

Interaction Design

Considering design as form and function in context allows products to be seen as objects; a meaning-led approach extends its connection with users. Buchanan's third order of design moves from object to interaction, an approach that embraces human-centred design. In these accounts, the user is a resource and design is focused on understanding and delivering what users want. It sees designers as part of a wider group of agents in the process of co-production or co-creation. It also accounts for changes in understanding the process of designing, suggesting that we are constituted in relation to the world not only as thinking subjects but also as bodily beings (Schön 1983).

With interaction design, the designer becomes an actor who is able to listen to users and facilitate the discussion about the design process. This approach can be communitarian in focus or applied to individual service encounters (e.g. an individual patient in a hospital) in which the user is a bringer of capability. In service design, where users are engaged in the design process and outcomes, a basic requirement is to find a balance between what designers try to fix and what is to be left free.

To account for this interactivity between design and user, models of user-engaging design have emerged. Sanders and Stappers (2008) define two mindsets: 'expert', in which users are subjects and reactive informers; and 'participatory', where the users are partners and active co-creators. User-centred design is therefore distinguished from participatory design by the active engagement of the user. Participatory co-design sees designers creating solutions with people from a community and recognises that local value chain actors can leverage local knowledge. It can also lead to innovations that may be better adapted to their context and be more likely to be adopted, since local people have invested resources in their creation (Brown 2008). With co-creation, users have a proactive role and should be involved at every stage of design development and as early as possible (Keränen et al. 2013).

These perspectives define a design agenda for PMDs. Designing has moved from a focus on the designer's creativity directed towards an object to a broader range of concerns and activities. The ability to relate form and functionality to products remains an important but not an exclusive aspect of designing. It is difficult both to design and to appreciate design without paying attention to its meaning. Moreover, the designer as facilitator or force for change, working with users and participants, has expanded the role and possibilities for design. The next section further develops these perspectives on user participation and cocreation, and by focusing on the design of PMDs in the health sector, it introduces wellbeing as an objective of participative design.

Design for Care

Contemporary healthcare is characterised by an increasing array of medical devices for diagnosis, prevention, monitoring and treatment of disease (World Health Organisation 2003; EC 2001) and more specifically the management of injuries and control of conception (Global Harmonzation Task Force 2005). Wearable medical devices placed on our bodies play a role in our personal and intimate worlds, influencing our everyday lives and self-perception. Faulkner (2008, p. 27) discusses the depth and reach of their influence and explains that:

> Medical devices enter into our intimate and family relationships, into our understandings of health and disease, our values and beliefs, our practices of looking after our own health, as well as our experience of healthcare systems and healthcare professionals' work.

As a subset of medical devices, wearable medical devices are worn objects. They are characterised as autonomous, usually non-invasive artefacts that are located on the body to perform their medical purpose (Fotiadis 2006). This requires devices to operate in a range of social, non-medical settings for a variety of activities in which the wearer may engage in their everyday lives, and to be wearable in all these settings.

Further research has focused upon orthoses as a specific form of wearable medical devices, also known as splints, braces and supports (Fess et al. 2004). Generally, splints function to immobilise, restrain and support the joint and are designed by hand therapists and occupational therapists based in hospitals. One important issue affecting the efficacy of splints is the low rate of patient adherence to their prescribed use. As found with other PMDs, whilst many people choose to wear these objects as prescribed, for others it is evident that the design of wearable medical devices within the traditional biomedical model creates arte-facts that can lead to low adherence and dissatisfaction.

There are a number of reasons for low splint adherence. Paterson's (2013) review of the literature identified important problems with wear-ability, including: inappropriateness for the patient's condition; diffi-culty to remove and put on; issues with comfort and fit; hygiene; and perceptions of both impracticality and undesirability. Furthermore, splints may be socially and emotionally unacceptable. Other research-ers have reported issues of style, aesthetics and cosmesis affecting patient adherence (McKee and Rivard 2011). In order to address this, McKee and Rivard suggest that an approach which situates health within a biopsychosocial model might be a productive direction for orthotic intervention.

The biopsychosocial model of health (BPS; Engel 1977) encompasses psychological, social and biological factors. In addition, we might think of health as an ability to adapt and to self-manage (Huber et al. 2011). More specifically, health requires 'the sufficient competence of a per-son to cope through self-regulation with any stressful disturbance on every system level' (Egger, 2013, p. 26). In these ways, it challenges the dominant biomedical model, with its focus upon the biological body (Fox 2012). By adopting a personalised treatment approach towards the patient, the BPS model provides versatility for care and opens up a broader consideration of wellbeing within the design process.

These understandings are also taken up in participatory medicine, a form of co-operative healthcare in which patients, healthcare profes-sionals, caregivers and other stakeholders are actively involved in the management of an individual's health (Gruman and Smith 2009). In this model, an important factor is the relationship between the health-care professional and patient and the sharing of decision-making with the aim of patient concordance rather than compliance (Mullen 1997).

Table 11.1 Fifteen guiding principles proposed by McKee and Rivard (2011)

• A patient or client- centred approach	• Optimise comfort
• Psychosocial factors	• Cosmesis
• Optimise body structure and function	• Convenience
• Enable activity and participation	• Use 'less is more' approach
• Well engineered	• Provide education
• Optimise usability	• Monitor and modify
• Provide choice	• Evaluate outcomes
• Minimise harm	

This move towards participatory, personalised medicine is similar to the shift of focus from object-centred to experience-centred design (Sleeswijk Visser 2009). It highlights a design for care approach and its effectiveness through participation in the design of new services and medical devices (Jones 2013).

McKee and Rivard (2011) propose fifteen guiding principles to undertake such a design process (Table 11.1). These support McDonagh's (2006) assertions that there is a need for a balanced approach to both functionality and supra-functionality, which is achieved by designing with rather than for people (Weightman and McDonagh 2003).

Although these principles are far reaching, they do not consider the fundamental reasons why people choose to wear objects on their bodies. In this respect, a craft sensibility firstly provides insights into the cultural and personal significances of wearing objects through the exploration of material and process (White and Steel 2007). Secondly, this approach extends the understanding that the experience of wearing a medical device is similar to the experience of wearing jewellery:

> …the sensation of touch on the body is pre-eminent, but movement and gesture, signal and message also become active participants in a web of visual, physical and psychological elements. (Watkins 1999)

This intimate relationship between the worn object and the wearer's sense of identity and wellbeing is often overlooked by research into wearable medical devices. For George Simmel, the jewellery-object performs or communicates the wearer's identity to others by singling 'out its wearer, whose self-feeling it embodies and increases at the cost of others' (Frisby and Featherstone 1997, p.207). Whilst personal identities and their maintenance are integral to individual wellbeing (Bostrom and Sandberg 2011), the implications for wearable medical devices and patient adherence are considerable and deserve further consideration. Contemporary jewellery provides a framework in which to locate and investigate their design.

Contemporary jewellery design is a movement originating from the 1950s that considers and challenges the themes and properties of jewellery (Skinner 2013). It acknowledges that the relationships between object, maker, wearer and viewer provide continual communication and interpretation of aspects such as identity and cultural values through semiotics and material use (Mazumdar 2014). As a craft, contemporary jewellery can be presented as both an approach and an attitude (Adamson 2007), and it is posited that this approach provides a new direction for co-design and design for care creating the therapeutic jewellery solutions described in the case study later in the chapter.

The similarities of jewellery and wearable medical devices begin with their characteristic of being worn or carried on the body, where they can play 'an active part in constituting the particular experience of the self, in determining what the self is' (Miller 2010, p. 40). Whilst jewellery is crafted to appear distinctive and (in the case of bespoke pieces) also crafted to the needs and desires of the individual client, the wearable medical device is designed with a medical aura that only considers the medical needs of the client. The value of the medical device is measured by its ability to restore or maintain the biomedical health of its wearer, whereas it is the emotional and material value of jewellery that is often the focus of wearability and meaning for the wearer.

Between wearable medical objects and jewellery lies an intersection in which therapeutic jewellery is located. This space enables the creation of therapeutic jewellery, a hybrid object that applies a craft approach to develop wearable objects that are aesthetically pleasing and emotionally engaging, potentially leading to improved adherence. In this respect, biomedical considerations are still important but the psychosocial aspects of wellbeing are also incorporated into their design. This therapeutic approach embraces a holistic consideration of what it means to be human and to wear objects on the body, alongside medical objectives.

A synergy of design approaches that encourage the wearer to adhere to their prescription may thus be proposed. These approaches are embedded within the biopsychosocial model, in which biomedical diagnosis is just one aspect and participatory design is an integral part. This model is interwoven into a design for care approach, where craft is acknowledged as a vehicle to construct meaning and offer dignity to people's lives. We locate the participatory and craft design of splints and other wearable medical devices within a contemporary jewellery framework that focuses on the exploration of the richly human aspects of health and wearability. The impact of wearable medical devices on the wearer can then be considered through the identification of the qualities and associations of both jewellery and wearable medical devices, thus highlighting the limitations of traditional medical device design. Here, a third approach (co-design for care) is developed to create therapeutic jewellery, hybrid objects incorporating the philosophies of craft and medical knowledge. As Jones (2013) explains:

> Designing for care brings a holistic and systemic design perspective to the complex problems of healthcare. Services have been already improved by designing better artefacts, communications, and environments. What is missing is the mindset of professional care in designing for people, practitioners, and societies. (p. 8)

Consequently, these design approaches incorporate a caring design ethic (Jones 2013) towards health-promoting artefacts. The ethic requires designers to adopt the role of healthcare professionals and to consider how design processes and outputs best promote all aspects of patients' wellbeing. This ethic is promoted through the selection of participatory and empathic design research methods to increase an understanding of people's everyday lives. Empathic design enquires about lived experience, with the aim of understanding the people's authentic perspective (McDonagh 2006). By using methods that develop empathy, the designer is able 'to become closer to the user through respectful curiosity, genuine understanding, and suspension of judgment' (McDonagh et al. 2009, p. 310). Participant engagement in generating design solutions arises from the personal crafting of objects. Their qualities, functionality, comfort and so on, when combined with their meanings, provide exemplars of processes and outputs that are readily accessible to others. Furthermore, data regarding the supra-functional needs of the user, which include the emotional, spiritual, social aspirational and cultural aspects of relationships with products, allow for object design to enable people to engage with objects at both rational and emotional levels (Chapman 2005).

These participatory processes help to overcome problems of self-selection bias, where the decision to participate can be perceived as an opportunity to promote awareness of interests, activism or 'setting the record straight'. The use of craft techniques focuses participants on the creative and aesthetic qualities of the designed orthotic object, as a means of engaging with the process of personalisation rather than its verbalisation. Further, they help to overcome problems of tokenism, or perfunctory engagement with a small number of patients. Participative design necessarily requires small groups and purposive sampling techniques that can be applied to specific medical conditions.

These perspectives also demonstrate how healthcare is evolving through the adoption of a design for care ethos. The growing acceptance of patients as equal partners creates an environment for design interventions and enables the holistic design of medical objects. In the context of wearable medical devices, therapeutic jewellery is a co-designed person-centric health device. These aspects are explained more fully in the following case study, which demonstrates generative design methods to inform and inspire therapeutic jewellery design to meet the needs of patients.

Case Study: The Craft of Wearable Wellbeing

The case study presented here was a practice-based project to research the design of therapeutic jewellery. This project was informed by the designer-researcher's experience of wearing orthoses to manage hEDS-ht. These orthoses were worn long term to manage pain and to immobilise the joints after dislocation or soft-tissue injury. Orthoses are commonly used by hEDS-ht patients to manage the condition, alongside a prescribed physiotherapy regime. This entails wearing a range of different orthoses for the affected joints throughout the day and night and over a lifetime, for the range of acute and chronic issues that the hEDS-ht patient experiences.

The research agenda hypothesised that designing within the biomedical model results in wearable medical devices with a medical register and low patient adherence. Consequently, a biopsychosocial design model was proposed for the design of a new hybrid artefact: therapeutic jewellery that promotes all dimensions of the wearer's wellbeing.

The case study synthesises design approaches, using principles of generative design, participative design, contemporary jewellery design and digital fabrication within a biopsychosocial health framework. The aims were to explore methods, practices and artefacts that support design for care processes in order to improve the design and services of these objects. This account focuses upon three aspects of the design process: the development of co-design methods for the PMD; implications for design arising from a hybrid design approach; and the conceptualisation of a co-designed orthosis.

Co-Designing for Care

Generative design research is carried out at the front end of the design process (Sanders and Stappers 2012). The project comprised a series of elements; the objectives and rationale for each activity are outlined in Table 11.2. An initial scoping exercise was promoted by HMSA (Hypermobility Syndromes Association) to its membership, where they were directed to respond to via email or social media (Twitter

Table 11.2 Elements of the research project

Element	Description and instructions	Objectives
Scoping study	Questionnaire Series of 9 questions regarding wearing orthoses Further discussions on Facebook and by email	To test hypothesis that wearers are dis-satisfied with available designs, which leads to low adherence To explore themes arising from the data To generate information to inform workshop
Sensitising pack	Sent 2 weeks before workshop Workbook that includes short daily activities Photography tasks Questions regarding the wearing of orthoses Clay model of something precious to the participant	To immerse workshop participants in making observations and reflections To allow participants to address feelings and thoughts about topic To gather further data regarding the experience of wearing orthoses
Workshop exercise A:	**Create a collage box** showing participant's wellbe-ing experience. Using a cardboard box template, choose from 100 images (both abstract and concrete) and 20 words (expressing feelings and emotions) to make a col-lage covering four sides of the box Individuals to share story with the group	To generate data that: Improves designer-researcher empathy Informs aesthetic decisions Explores meaning-making
Workshop exercise B:	**3D model of dream device of the future** Choosing from the range of crafting materi-als provided, to create a model of your dream wearable medical device Participants to share each model with the group	To generate data that: Informs the further design process Identifies key themes and issues regard-ing orthoses Increases empathy

(continued)

Table 11.2 (continued)

Element	Description and instructions	Objectives
Analysis of data	Thematic analysis Metaphor analysis: Image schemata (Johnson 1990) Visual analysis Methodological triangulation	To analyse data: Note patterns, themes & clusters Making metaphors Making contrasts/comparisons To assume a coherent understanding of the data
Design concept	Devise possible ways forward based on analysis of data: Design artefacts: Scanned CAD of wrist Collection of wrist splints as therapeutic jewellery: 1. Desktop 3D printed 2. Traditional jewellery techniques: using silver and wood 3. SLS 3D printed Web-based digital health project	To explore the possibilities that technologies offer to improve the design of orthoses and the design process for recipients To develop a range of wrist splints within contemporary jewellery framework To explore idea of digital health project with open source designs available

and a Facebook project page open to comments). This generated data from respondents that supported the research hypothesis, and which informed the design of a sensitising pack and a workshop. The aim of the sensitising pack was to allow participants to explore the scope of the topic and consisted of a workbook with short daily tasks that included taking photos of objects and settings, and describing aspects of their personal splint use.

This process was subsequently developed in a workshop, where participants became co-partners with the designer-researcher. A group of between four and eight participants enabled the workshop facilitators to pay attention to every individual (Sleeswijk Visser et al. 2005). Seven women were recruited for the workshop with the support of HMSA. These women all have hEDS-ht and long-term experience of wearing orthoses. They were motivated to take part due to their dissatisfaction with wearing orthoses and their desire to engage with the design process in order to create devices with more wearability. The workshop was women-only in order to focus on wearable solutions that incorporated notions of adornment for women, and to create a safe space for women to discuss sensitive issues (i.e., body image). At the time of the workshop, half of the participants were working whilst the other half were medically retired due to hEDS-ht. The women ranged in age from the twenties to the early sixties. This research was seen as the opening trial in a series of studies to research the experiences of patients with different medical conditions who wear wearable medical devices and to investigate patient involvement throughout the design process.

The principle behind generative techniques is to allow people to make designerly artefacts and individually share stories about their objects (Sleeswijk Visser et al. 2005). Two exercises were organised for the workshop, both using craft-based representational strategies. Participants individually created a collage and a 3D model that they then shared with the group. This employed a craft approach on the basis that craft and art practice allows for the ideas of participants to be embodied and given form in the model-making process (Sullivan 2006), and on the basis that 'by connecting people on emotional and visceral levels, artistic forms of representation facilitate empathy' (Leavy 2015,

p. 14). The qualitative data generated was then analysed to inspire and inform the concept design of orthotic wrist splints.

The first exercise generated data regarding participants' experiences of their own wellbeing and illness. Participants made an individual collage in a cardboard box form, using a collection of 100 images and 20 words to describe their own feelings and experiences towards wellbeing. On completion, they shared their models and personal narratives with the group. Collage is a widely used technique in qualitative research (Leavy 2015), helping the collage-maker access intuitive knowledge and enabling communication on a metaphorical level (Butler-Kisber and Poldma 2010). The second exercise entailed participants considering their 'dream health device' and producing a 3D model, again sharing their models with the group. This enabled them to explore solutions for orthoses and accessed their 'tacit' knowledge (Polanyi 2002) regarding these artefacts.

Implications for Design from the Participatory Workshop

Themes identified in the scoping exercise and sensitising pack were supported through analysis of the data generated by the participants' 3D models of splints within the workshops. These data included the transcripts of participants' discussions regarding their models and the researcher's visual analysis and assessment. In discussions, participants demonstrated their expertise regarding wearability by identifying the design factors that influence the wearability of orthoses. These were identified as: fit; function; style; aesthetics; materials; method of making; emotional engagement and meaning (Fig. 11.1). Each of these factors impacts upon the wearer's adherence to the device and needs to be addressed if wearability and adherence are to be improved.

Participants felt conflicted between wearing orthoses and feeling that these artefacts were socially undesirable. As one respondent commented:

> I don't want to be defined and judged by 'granny beige' splints and surgical looking supports... I am a young woman who happens to have a disability - that's a side note. I also happen to have a very definite sense of style and that WILL translate to the very things that are meant to make my life easier and better, so help me!

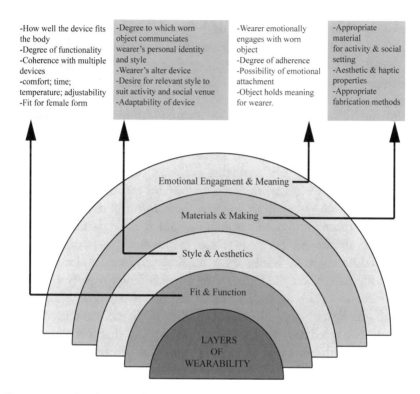

-How well the device fits the body
-Degree of functionality
-Coherence with multiple devices
-comfort; time; temperature; adjustability
-Fit for female form

-Degree to which worn object communciates wearer's personal identity and style
-Wearer's alter device
-Desire for relevant style to suit activity and social venue
-Adaptability of device

-Wearer emotionally engages with worn object
-Degree of adherence
-Possibility of emotional attachment
-Object holds meaning for wearer.

-Appropriate material for activity & social setting
-Aesthetic & haptic properties
-Appropriate fabrication methods

Emotional Engagment & Meaning

Materials & Making

Style & Aesthetics

Fit & Function

LAYERS OF WEARABILITY

Fig. 11.1   Design factors influencing orthotic wearability

Participants were very clear about the effect of wearing orthoses. One commented on finding a device that she could wear to a social occasion: 'For 2 hours I regained my "mojo" and felt like me'. Another summed up more negative experiences:

> Generally, very little thought goes into them in my experience, for people who have to wear them constantly. Sure, if you break your wrist and need to wear a splint for six weeks you can put up with it being hot and sweaty and looking horrible, but not if you have to wear it day in and day out.

Their awareness of material properties of objects worn on the body highlighted issues of breathability and thermoregulation, with many comments mirroring one participant's observation that 'the material not being hot and clammy would be good, making it look more like an accessory than a splint, and breathable'. Aesthetic qualities were also commented on. Whilst Velcro was seen as useful, it was also disliked because it 'catches on things, ruining the splints or other clothing and scratching skin'.

The workshop generated a range of insightful data that demonstrated this group's negative perceptions regarding the poor wearability of orthoses and the accompanying negative impact this had on their sense of wellbeing. Through participants' accounts, current orthoses emerge as 'ugly', 'sweaty', 'unstylish', impractical and difficult to use over the long term. Both cosmetic aspects and the comfort of day-to-day use are addressed through such understandings, which made participants unenthusiastic about, and less likely to use, the medically prescribed orthoses they had been given. Whilst these medical orthoses may 'work' physiologically to support the joints, if their poor design negatively impacts on wellbeing and frequency of use, their overall success in improving health might be more questionable. The feedback from participants points to a need for design to develop devices that people can easily engage with emotionally and that they can perceive as meaningful in their lives. To this end, designers need to consider how it looks and feels on the body, how it makes the wearer feels, and how it fits into their world. Materiality is the key in this respect, with a strong need for materials that perform well on the body and do not create the sweatiness and smell that some complained about. Whilst people want the device to function appropriately and fit well, the important design aspects for these artefacts are those relating to more intangible wearability factors of personal style, emotional engagement and meaning, and it is in these areas where contemporary jewellery design can propose stylised solutions. Orthosis design should be considered in the context of self-identity and style. Consumer behaviour in fashion retailing demonstrates not only instrumental intentions to purchase but also emotional ones, in which choice, contemporary styling and endorsement through many media have major roles. In brief, the findings highlight the importance of holistic solutions and a transdisciplinary approach to orthotic design.

Developing Co-Designed Orthoses

The research subsequently moved into the conceptualisation phase (Sanders and Stappers 2012), generating a series of relevant concepts inspired by the research insights. The designer-researcher approached the design of therapeutic jewellery in an emergent manner, engaging with the source material through a reflective practice that explored design through drawing, models and the investigation of material qualities. She began by creating a collage using those images and words most used by the participants. The themes of 'freedom' and the ability to choose paths were important to workshop participants and suggested their desire for a range of choices when it came to orthoses available for them. It was decided to explore how technologies could best be employed for this purpose whilst addressing the layers of wearability, and, importantly, considering how these artefacts could promote the emotional engagement and meaning that jewellery ideally creates in the wearer. The two popular images that participants used in their collages were 'Amazon Warrior' and 'Wonder Woman', and the frequent uses of the word 'strength' were in direct opposition to the feelings of loss, chaos and brokenness that participants experienced. These were used playfully by the designer-researcher to inspire and generate designs to be worn by the two archetypes of Amazon Warrior and Wonder Woman in the twenty-first century. The image of a gift proved popular, and the maker considered how the orthoses could be considered, similar to jewellery, as gifts. These approaches to the data demonstrate craft functioning as a vehicle to construct meaning, whilst offering substance and grace to people's lives (Metcalf 2002).

A series of wrist-splints-as-therapeutic-jewellery were then devised, embracing a range of digital and analogue technologies used in contemporary jewellery making. As a creative and craft process, the designer employed 3D technology and collaborations with silversmiths and a cabinetmaker to achieve designs using 3D printing materials alongside a collection using silver and wood. Techniques include measuring the wrist dimensions and fabricating the device using traditional bench techniques, where silver is manipulated using rolling mills and hammers. Digital technologies were used, including scanning the wrist into a CAD programme and designing the device directly onto the wrist model, and then 3D printing the device. The first collection of designs was fabricated by a desktop 3D printer (Fig. 11.2) to demonstrate the possibilities of using domestically available technologies, whilst a second collection used SLS 3D technology. A third collection was created using traditional jewellery materials such as silver and wood (Fig. 11.3). The devices were custom-fitted to the designer-researcher's own wrist. The ability to provide a perfect fit by both digital and analogue methods demonstrated the ease by which personalised orthotics can be fabricated.

In addition, a digital health project was proposed, offering a web-based service for wearers of orthoses. Open designs will be displayed within a digital library on this site for others to access for printing and to further develop the designs. The project would work as an open design project where the designer becomes 'a database designer, a meta-designer, not designing objects, but shaping a design space in which unskilled users can access user-friendly environments in which they can design their own objects' (De Mul 2011, p. 36). The approach includes

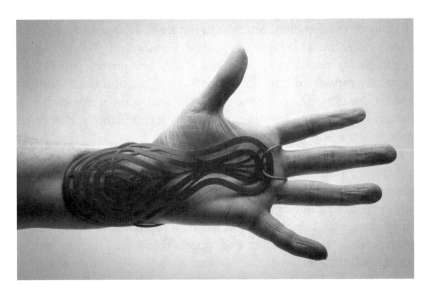

Fig. 11.2   Fresh Embrace, desktop 3D printed orthosis (Photo credit: J. Senior)

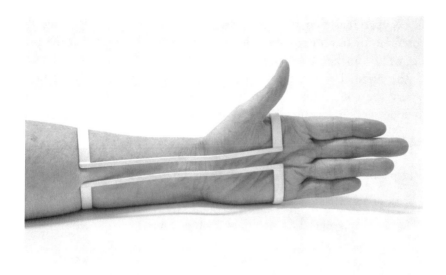

Fig. 11.3   Minimum wrist device (silver) (Photo credit: J. Senior)

the use of scanning technology that can scan body parts and import the data into a CAD programme. Designs can be then adjusted for an exact fit for each person with the wearer also choosing from a range of materials and finishes.

The design of these artefacts with craft sensibility seeks to provide functionality along with an ability to express human values (Risatti 2009). As such, the crafted object is both theorised and personalised through a radical and innovative process (Yair et al. 2001; Adamson 2010), and embraces a definition of contemporary jewellery in which ideas are served by materials and skills (Skinner 2013). Furthermore, the digital health project empowers patients to co-create personalised artefacts, whilst remaining engaged in the design and production processes.

Reviews of the collections have been positive with The Orthotics Campaign (2016) commenting that the work is 'exciting and creative'. When the 3D printed work was exhibited, viewers recorded how 'stylish', 'funk' and 'upbeat' the devices were, with some asking if they could be worn without a medical prescription. Healthcare professionals such as occupational therapists also responded positively, recognising the potential for transdisciplinary design teams with the hope that the project will be further developed.

The original research respondents and participants were invited to review the collections, and their comments endorsed the potential of such devices. One commented:

> Having some sort of control over the devices, choices, supports etc. that
>
> help improve my quality of living daily gives me back a sense of self and
>
> sense of respect and, if people have that, they are less likely to become
>
> depressed and spiral downwards physically and mentally.

Another observed that the personalised approach was empowering:

> Thank you so much for this, I'm a HUGE advocate of empowering
>
> people through choices and being a disabled young woman, I have
>
> felt 'weak' and 'visible' (and also 'invisible' at times) when out and about in
>
> what can sometimes seem like a huge, flashing 'look at me' set of NHS
>
> beige-ness.

These comments are representative of the positive feedback that was received. Indeed, the only negative comments related to personal tastes and device needs, which further support the need for a person-centric approach that incorporates the full range of wearability factors. This reflects the need for a shift in perspective for orthosis design away from a medical model to a social model of prescription (Pullin 2009).

Co-Design for Care

The design for care process employed by this research develops a therapeutic design approach that becomes a new and powerful addition to co-design. It presents possibilities for enhancing patients' agency in their healthcare by enabling them to articulate their expertise in wearing medical objects and by engaging them in applying tacit knowledge to craft objects that address the eight layers of wearability (Table 11.2). Creating objects that incorporate qualities of jewellery such as preciousness and desirability may be particularly attractive to women, but its focus on detail and the opportunities to create personalised and meaningful objects that people want to wear has cross-gender appeal. Therapeutic design provides new processes for participation building upon the co-design approach and foregrounding the importance of wellbeing as an outcome. This approach offers solutions to achieving the service criteria defined by the Associate Parliamentary Limb Loss Group (2011) for comfort, choice and cosmesis (the preservation, restoration or enhancement of physical appearance). Since research respondents were concerned about the lack of fast and efficient access to 'right first time' devices, a service provision that employs cheap and effective digital technologies to fabricate personalised solutions could well address these issues. This approach is supported by the Orthotics campaign (2014). Interestingly, there are also developments in the private sector, such as Andiamo (2016), set up by e-patients, who aim to deliver a 3D printed medically effective orthosis within 1 week, alongside an advanced clinical service.

PMDs provide a valuable focus for the exploration of design principles and practices, demonstrating an established commitment to functionality whilst increasing understanding of engagement with the user. Design aesthetics have been discussed in terms of form, in particular for products and their relationship with functionality. In commercial design, products must always have sales appeal; appearances are targeted at markets of potential consumers who have awareness of a very wide range of well-designed products. PMDs can draw on this commercial appeal, not least as publicly funded healthcare gives way to more mixed models of private–public partnerships. Nevertheless, they challenge notions of form, style, and design as both process and outcome in order to stimulate reflection on the increasingly diverse processes of design. Creating or facilitating meanings of PMDs by their users is an important and neglected consideration in their design. It extends the designer–object relationship into one of the co-creative processes with users. Established models of PMD design contribute to reduced wearer adherence; consequently, alternative approaches are desirable. The case study presented above demonstrates how a biopsychosocial model can be used to contextualise new ways of designing orthotics with positive outcomes. It highlights the personal experience of the medical device, how it is sensed, and its contribution to social wearability and identity. As a result, participation in PMD design enables patients to be more aware of their wellbeing, adhere to the use of devices and be more engaged in the personalisation of their healthcare. We suggest that design, as well as use, allows individualised health technologies to become 'personal'.

Note

1. All workshop material used in this chapter was gained with informed consent and is used with permission.

References

Adamson, G. (2007). *Thinking through craft*. Oxford: Berg.

Adamson, G. (2010). *The craft reader*. Oxford: Berg.

Andiamo. (2016). Andiamo user-centred children's orthotics. Available at: www.andiamo.io [Accessed May 01, 2016].

Associate Parliamentary Limb Loss Group. (2011). Patient led orthotic services with the support of this users charter (Orthotics Charter). CES Available at: http://nsoc.org.uk/evidence/Orthotics+Charter+2011+apllg+Aug+11.pdf [Accessed May 10, 2016].

Bostrom, N., & Sandberg, A. (2011). The future of identity, report. *Commissioned by the UK's Government Office for Science*. Available at: http://www.nickbostrom.com/views/identity.pdf [Accessed December 15, 2015].

Brown, T. (2008). Design thinking. *Harvard Business Review, 86*(6), 84–92.

Buchanan, R. (2001). Designing and the new learning. *Design Issues, 17*(4), 3–23.

Butler-Kisber, L., & Poldma, T. (2010). The power of visual approaches in qualitative inquiry: The use of collage making and concept mapping in experiential. *Journal of Research Practice, 6*(2), 18.

Chapman, J. (2005). *Emotionally durable design*. London: Earthscan.

De Mul, J. (2011). Redesigning. In B. Van Abel, L. Evers, R. Klaassen, & P. Troxler (Eds.), *Open design now* (pp. 34–39). Amsterdam: BIS.

Dreyfus, H. (1967). *Designing for people*. New York NY: Paragraphic Books.

EC. (2001). *Guidelines for the classification of medical devices*. Brussels: European Commission.

Egger, J. W. (2013). Biopsychosocial Medicine and Health – the body mind unity theory and its dynamic definition of health. *Psychologische Medizin, 24*(1), 24–29.

Engel, G. L. (1977). The need for a new medical model: A challenge for biomedicine. *Science, New Series, 196*(4286), 129–136.

Faulkner, A. (2008). *Medical technology into healthcare and society: A sociology of devices, innovation and governance*. Basingstoke: Palgrave Macmillan.

Fess, E. E., Gettle, K. S., Philips, C. A., & Janson, J. R. (2004). *Hand and upper extremity splinting: Principles and methods*. St. Louis, MI: Mosby Inc.

Fotiadis, D. I., Glaros, C., & Likas, A. (2006). Wearable medical devices. *Wiley Encyclopedia of Biomedical Engineering*. Chichester: Wiley-Interscience.

Fox, N. (2012). *The body*. Cambridge: Polity Press.

Frisby, D., & Featherstone, M. (1997). *Simmel on culture: Selected writings*. London: Sage.

Glanze, W. D., Anderson, K., & Anderson, L. E. (1990). *Mosby's medical, nursing, and allied health dictionary*. St. Louis, MI: Mosby.

Global Harmonization Task Force. (2005). Information Document Concerning the Definition of the Term "Medical Device" SG1/NO29R11. http://www.imdrf.org/docs/ghtf/final/sg1/technical-docs/ghtf-sg1-n29r16-2005-definition-medical-device-050520.pdf [Accessed 12th January 2016].

Golubnitschaja, O., Kinkorova, J., & Costigliola, V. (2014). Predictive, preventive and as the hardcore of 'Horizon 2020': EPMA position paper. *EPMA Journal, 5*(6). Available from http://www.epmajournal.com/content/5/1/6 [Accessed August 12, 2016].

Gruman, J., & Smith, C. W. (2009). Why the journal of participatory medicine? *Journal of Participatory Medicine., 1*(1), 2.

HEC (Health Economics Consortium). (2009). *Orthotic service in the NHS: Improving service provision*. York: University of York.

Huber, M., Knottnerus, J. A., Green, L., van der Horst, H., Jadad, A. R., Kromhout, D., et al. (2011). How should we define health? *British Medical Journal, 343,* d4163.

Johnson, M. (1990). *The body in the mind*. Chicago, IL: University of Chicago Press.

Jones, P. (2013). *Design for care: Innovating healthcare experience*. New York: Rosenfeld Media.

Keränen, K., Dusch, B., Ojasalo, K., & Moultrie, J. (2013). Co-creation patterns : Insights from a collaborative service tool. *In the Proceedings of The Cambridge Academic Design Management Conference*. Cambridge: University of Cambridge.

Krippendorff, K. (1989). On the essential contexts of artifacts or on the proposition that "is making sense (of things)". *Design Issues, 5*(2), 9–38.

Krippendorff, K. (2006). *The semantic turn: A new foundation for design*. Boca Raton, FL: CRC Press.

Lambert, S. (1993). *Form follows function. Design in the 20th century*. London: Victoria and Albert Museum.

Leavy, P. (2015). *Method meets art: Arts-based research practice*. New York: Guilford Publications.

Llewellyn, D. (2010). *The first lady of mulberry walk*. Leicester: Troubadour.

Mazumdar, P. (2014). Understanding surfaces. On jewellery and identity. Lecture (March 16, 2014) at Die Neue Sammlung Pinakothek Der Moderne Munich, in collaboration with Arnoldsche Art Publishers.

McDonagh, D. (2006). Empathic design: Emerging design research methodologies. *PhD dissertation*. Loughborough: Loughborough University.

McDonagh, D., Thomas, J., Chen, S., He, J. J., Hong, Y. S., Kim, Y., Zhang, Z., et al. (2009). Empathic : Disability + relevant design. *In the Proceedings of 8th European Academy of Design Conference April*. 310. Aberdeen: The Robert Gordon University.

McKee, P. R., & Rivard, A. (2011). Biopsychosocial approach to orthotic intervention. *Journal of Hand Therapy: Official Journal of the American Society of Hand Therapists, 24*(2), 155–162.

Metcalf, B. (2002). Contemporary craft: A brief overview. In J. Johnson (Ed.), *Exploring contemporary craft: History, theory & critical writing*. Toronto: Coach House Books and Harbourfront Center.

Miller, D. (2010). *Stuff*. Cambridge: Polity.

Mullen, P. D. (1997). Compliance becomes concordance. *BMJ, 314*(7082), 691.

National Institutes of Health. (2008). Biennial report of the national institutes of health, fiscal years, 2006–2007. U.S. Department of Health and Human Services. Available at: https://www.report.nih.gov/biennialreport0607/NIH_BR_Chapter1.pdf [Accessed May 10, 2016].

NHS England. (2015). *Improving the quality of orthotics services in England.* London: NHS England.

Orthotics Campaign. (2014). Factors that affect the patient experience of NHS orthotics care ONLINE. Available at: https://www.england.nhs.uk/wp-content/uploads/2015/11/orthcs-rep-attach-1.pdf [Accessed November 25, 2016].

Orthotics Campaign. (2016). Personal communication. February 11.

Parsons, G. (2016). *The philosophy of design.* Cambridge: Polity Press.

Paterson, A. (2013). Digitisation of the splinting process: Exploration and evaluation of a computer aided approach to support additive manufacture. *Doctoral Dissertation.*

Polanyi, M. (2002). *Personal knowledge: Towards a post-critical philosophy.* London: Routledge.

Pullin, G. (2009). *Design meets disability.* Cambridge, MA: MIT Press.

Risatti, H. (2009). *A theory of craft: Function and aesthetic expression.* Charlotte, CA: University of North Carolina Press.

Sanders, E. B.-N., & Stappers, P. J. (2008). Co-creation and the new landscapes of design: *CoDesign, 4*(1), 5–18.

Sanders, E. B.-N., & Stappers, P. J. (2012). *Convivial toolbox: Generative research for the front end of design.* Amsterdam: BIS publishers.

Schön, D. (1983). *The reflective practitioner: How professionals think in action.* Farnham: Ashgate.

Simon, H. A. (1969). *The sciences of the artificial.* Cambridge, MA: MIT Press.

Skinner, D. (Ed.). (2013). *Contemporary jewelry in perspective.* New York: Lark Jewelry & Beading.

Sleeswijk Visser, F. S. (2009). Bringing the Everyday Life of People into Design. *PhD Dissertation.* Delft: TU Delft.

Sleeswijk Visser, F. S., Stappers, P. J., van der Lugt, R., & Sanders, E. B. (2005). Contextmapping: Experiences from practice. *CoDesign, 1*(2), 119–149.

Sullivan, G. (2006). Artefacts as evidence within changing contexts. Working Papers in Art and Design 4, pp. 1–12.

Ulrich, K. T., & Eppinger, S. D. (2012). *Product design and development* (5th ed.). New York: McGraw Hill.

Utterback, J., Vedin, B.-A., Alvarez, E., Ekman, S., Sanderson, S. W., Tether, B., et al. (2006). *Design-inspired innovation.* London: Scientific.

Walsh, V. (1996). Design, innovation and the boundaries of the firm. *Research Policy, 25*(4), 502–529.

Watkins, D. (1999). *Design sourcebook: Jewellery.* London: New Holland.

Weightman, D., & McDonagh, D. (2003). People are doing it for themselves. *Proceedings of the 2003 International Conference on Designing Pleasurable Products and Interfaces.* 23–26 June. Pittsburgh USA, pp. 34–39.

White, H., & Steel, E. (2007). Agents of change: From collection to connection. *The Design Journal, 10*(2), 22–34.

World Health Organization. (2003). *Medical device regulations: Global overview and guiding principles.* Geneva: WHO Press.

Yair, K., Press, M., & Tomes, A. (2001). Crafting competitive advantage: Crafts knowledge as a strategic resource. *Design Studies, 22*(4), 377–394.

Part V
Conclusion

12

Quantified Lives and Vital Data: Some Concluding Remarks

Conor Farrington and Rebecca Lynch

Taken together, the preceding chapters demonstrate that the much-vaunted potential of technology in medical and wellness contexts is only part of the story. Personal medical devices (PMDs) do far more in practice than merely carrying out their intended technical functions. In addition to this, they produce lives that are both quantified and more tightly bound to medicine and medical monitoring, while also adding to, reframing and developing who we 'are' and what health and medicine may be. PMDs create dynamic bodies that 'live,' producing data that are both human and vital. These technologies not only tether us, but also enhance us; they are often mundane but can also be highly

C. Farrington (✉)
Cambridge Centre for Health Services Research, University of Cambridge, Cambridge, UK
e-mail: Cjtf2@medschl.cam.ac.uk

R. Lynch
London School of Hygiene and Tropical Medicine, University of London, London, UK
e-mail: Rebecca.Lynch@lshtm.ac.uk

© The Author(s) 2018
R. Lynch and C. Farrington (eds.), *Quantified Lives and Vital Data*,
Health, Technology and Society, https://doi.org/10.1057/978-1-349-95235-9_12

influential, opening up new possibilities even as they close down others. The papers in this collection illustrate and unpick these ideas in various ways, adopting different approaches and investigating different devices and contexts. Against the backdrop of this diversity, we end this collection by considering some of the cross-cutting themes that recur throughout the book, most notably a concern with the importance of looking at PMDs in their wider context and in use, rather than as historical, neutral, and disconnected objects. All chapters consider in various ways what these objects 'do' in the world and how they come into being or are 'made' (and themselves make other entities). PMDs are presented as shaping, and as being shaped by, intimate encounters between individuals and these technologies but also through more diverse meeting points: discussions on Internet forums and in MeetUp groups; programmes run by corporations for their employees; clinical researchers and trial participants; national and supra-national regulatory authorities; public health scientists; ethicists; designers, and patients and designers; and of course, engagements between researchers and their interlocutors. These encounters include interactions with other material entities—blood, muscles, skin, food, bicycles, testing equipment, and other technologies, for example—as well as with policies, scientific papers, discourses, and debates. As such, PMDs incorporate a range of other 'stuff' as well as a range of different practices.

Throughout the book, the entanglements of practice, power, positionality, and physicality in relation to PMDs are drawn out, together with a wider engagement with the connectedness of technologies, sociotechnical networks, and multiple kinds of users and stakeholders. Contributions acknowledge, and in some cases foreground, the wider organizational, institutional, supra-national, and policy contexts in which PMDs are situated, 'made' from, and utilised. Relationships between individuals, technology, and health appear in differing configurations, with some relationships appearing stronger or more foregrounded than others and at different times. These are not fixed relations, therefore, but dynamic and flexible relations, which are sometimes contradictory and amenable to change.

PMDs fit well into wider discourses about the need to further individualise medicine through newly available capacities, tailoring treatment, awareness of risk and provision of care according to individual biology. The growth of chronic diseases in contemporary societies has prompted an increased focus on health behavior and related risk factors, coalescing around a suggested need for individuals to self-manage and take responsibility for their own health. In turn, this has produced a focus on lifestyles as a key factor with regard to impacting on individuals' health status. Such lifestyles, and the bodies they produce, thereby become sites for monitoring and intervention. The papers in this collection furnish consideration of technologies and practices related to this illness-policy nexus, regarding the following: regulation of blood pressure monitors and coagulometers; the development of policy and evidence around e-cigarettes; self-management of Ehlers-Danlos Syndrome; and more widespread self-monitoring of individual activities such as cycling, running, and eating. While the two chapters that focus on diabetes technology (Hess and Farrington) focus on users with type 1 diabetes, an auto-immune condition, considerations presented by these authors are also pertinent when considering type 2 diabetes, which is one of the most prominent of chronic lifestyle-related diseases.

Many of the papers look at the data produced by these PMDs, focusing variously on how data are interpreted and by whom, and how these data might work with or against more embodied understandings of individuals' health, well-being, bodies, and sense of self. The data produced by such technologies may be related to personal experiences and sensemaking (sometimes undertaken with others), but is also linked to standardised 'norms' developed from other users, PMD producers, or wider population figures. Data may be personal and/or public and may be drawn on in different ways by different groups. Collectively, these papers raise questions about how the body and health are, or can be, 'known,' and whether such 'knowing' (and acting on this knowing) is an ethical duty. They demonstrate that data interpretation is never straightforward, being tied into many other concerns, practices, and material entities. They demonstrate, too, that these data are not neutral, objective, or 'independent' readings of biological processes, but, rather, actively emerge from quite specific encounters in which they are 'made.'

Related to this, many of the chapters consider PMDs 'outside the clinic'—e.g. PMDs used in the home, in everyday life and activities, or work. These use-contexts raise questions about where the medical field starts and ends. When steps walked in a day or kinds of food eaten are monitored by these health technologies, does this monitoring become a medical action? To what extent can PMDs be seen to contribute to arguments about the increasing medicalisation of our everyday lives? Whether the technologies themselves can be classed as straightforwardly 'medical' is also questioned by the chapters in this collection, particularly when issues of pleasure emerge. Pleasure is gained by women through ultrasound 'keepsakes' of their pregnancies, by smokers enjoying e-cigarettes, and by members of the Quantified Self movement using self-tracking technologies—but this does not contribute to these devices being classified as 'medical.' This leads to an interesting question regarding the relationship between pleasure and medicine: why are pleasurable things harder to fit into a medical framing? If walking and eating in particular ways (and monitoring them in particular ways, e.g. with PMDs) create not only health benefits but also pleasurable sensations, can they be considered as 'medical' actions? PMDs, therefore, may undermine (or at least give an alternative framing to) arguments of increased medicalisation in light of different ways in which health is 'done.' They not only trouble categories regarding who is/is not a patient, what health/illness may be, and what is medical/non-medical, but also invite new engagements in conceptualising self/non-self, public/private, ethical/non-ethical, natural/unnatural, and of course, user/non-user.

Collectively, the book contributes to growing attempts to explore, conceptualise, and interrogate PMDs in social, scientific, and medical settings while also underlining the diversity and complexity of relationships between people and medical technology. Our constructed portmanteau category of PMDs demonstrates that such technologies and relationships are always entangled with, and emerge through engagements with, wider social worlds. While there are a number of common themes across the chapters, only some of which have been discussed above, we have further drawn out three key points for consideration by those interested in developing further work in this area.

Through the chapters, PMDs can be seen to draw together different *connections*, emerging from and linking individuals with others, and with wider society and institutions. Who we think we are, how we think we are, and what we think medicine might be are all open to negotiation through PMDs, as new relations, boundaries, practices, and socialities may come into being while old ones are questioned and/ or sliced differently. In so doing, the chapters suggest that such concepts and clear boundaries are not as fixed or prescriptive as we might think. Notions of control, risk, and responsibility for health emerge also, as well as questions about the nature, interpretation, and use of data produced by different technologies. The key point to make here is that PMDs *do* things in use, often moving, relating to, producing, and incorporating a wide range of 'stuff' in unpredictable ways. The chapters collectively argue for grounded approaches to analysis of technologies *in practice*, alongside consideration of the other elements they work with, through and incorporate—i.e., the 'stuff' of those practices.

Secondly, and relating to this first point, technologies cannot be considered separately to the *practices* they are embedded within. PMDs, like other objects, are embedded in practices, spaces, times, and relationships, and do not stand apart from these. They are not separate from context but *are part of* context. The PMDs discussed in these chapters are situated—they are intimately connected to the wider circumstances in which the chapters describe them, and in fact become quite different things in different situations. For example, the insulin pumps in Hess' chapter are 'done' quite differently in different settings, even for the same person; the activity monitors used by Dudhwala's interlocutors enact different relationships and dynamics from those used by corporations in Till's contribution; and Lynch's chapter shows that e-cigarettes are helpful for reducing smoking for one group within public health and potentially harmful for another, with both sides drawing upon arguments and framings which may have very little to do with the material-semiotic practices of e-cigarette users themselves. Across the chapters, PMDs emerge as 'things' *through* their interactions in these different locations: it is not that the object stays the same and the context differs, but that the contexts *make* the PMDs themselves. This suggests that social analysis cannot examine PMDs as stand-alone objects outside context. Different situations produce different framings, relationships, power dynamics, and constructions.

Finally, PMDs are *intersections* where different institutions and sectors meet. Government, regulators, public and/or private health services, medical specialists, researchers and clinicians, commercial developers, interested individuals, employees and employers, citizens, patients, carers, advocacy groups, and designers are just some of the stakeholders who are brought together in differing configurations around PMDs within these chapters. As noted above, different situations produce different constructions, relationships, and power dynamics; what these objects are, how they are used, and what their meanings may be very different for these different groups, creating, reinforcing, and on some occasions (as Dudhwala's interlocutors might argue) equalising power relations. PMDs are not merely not-neutral, but are tools that are used in particular ways by and for particular benefits and with particular agendas in mind. From a health inequalities perspective, which emphasises the fact that poorer people generally have poorer health as well as more limited access to healthcare, it is important to recognize that many PMDs may further increase such disparities rather than (as is sometimes claimed) help to reduce them. We noted earlier that access to these technologies, and their usability and acceptability once in use, may vary widely. Owing to our focus on the broad UK context, the chapters in this collection do not explicitly consider local provision and use of such devices; nor do they discuss inequity experienced in low- and middle-income countries. Nevertheless, broader questions emerge throughout this collection about who benefits (and how) from PMD usage, and about what kinds of wider relations may be created, maintained, or disrupted through PMD use. For example, Smajdor and Stockl invite us to question the traditional privileges of medicine and how PMDs might alter these, including relationships between doctors and patients; Lynch illustrates the powerful constructions of people's relationships with objects within public health, constructions which are then turned into policy recommendations and health interventions; and Till sheds new light on the motives of corporations interested in the activity levels of their staff. In the context of sensemaking about biosensing bodies (Kragh-Furbo et al.), we might also consider variable familiarity with, and access to, Internet chat rooms, and the means through which the voices of some contributors are shut down while others become more dominant; and we might consider how, in the context of new technology trials (Farrington), the process of being recruited for such trials and subsequently performing as a 'good' participant (which may rely on qualities other than biomedical status) may set up particular dynamics between patients, clinicians, researchers, technology producers, and funders. The papers in this collection therefore connect PMDs to important wider structures, practices, dynamics, and relations, as discussed by Matthewman in his introductory chapter. So while the chapters argue for a consideration of PMDs in use and as situated within broader context, they also suggest an investigation of power dynamics and the wider consequences of the growth and development of PMDs. PMDs not only 'do' things in practice, but they do particular things for particular people. There is much scope for further investigation and nuanced unpicking of the power dynamics and relationships entangled with PMDs, and consequently this would be a fruitful direction for further work, particularly in considering how PMDs travel between contexts and different geographical scales from the local to the global. While this edited collection has presented some of the key issues and considerations for the dynamic and changing relationships between people, technology, and health through its focus on PMDs in the UK context, clearly PMDs, and the concepts and constructions they bring into focus, are part of far wider stories and relationships.

Through these chapters, we hope to have illustrated some of the complexities, questions, and opportunities for development in this expanding field. And through the conceptual bringing together of the personal, the medical, and the device, we have aimed to illuminate how these three aspects might work together, or indeed against each other, in particular ways and in particular use-contexts. This intersection, like PMDs themselves, is not fixed and unchanging, but provides a starting point for wider investigations—a path through which we might examine and give detailed accounts of quantified lives and vital data.

Index

Printed in the United States
By Bookmasters